A Parent's Guide to High-Functioning Autism Spectrum Disorder

How to Meet the Challenges and Help Your Child Thrive

SECOND EDITION

Sally Ozonoff
Geraldine Dawson
James C. McPartland

THE GUILFORD PRESS
New York   London

© 2015 The Guilford Press
A Division of Guilford Publications, Inc.
370 Seventh Avenue, Suite 1200, New York, NY 10001
www.guilford.com

Printed in the United States of America

Last digit is print number: 9   8   7

Library of Congress Cataloging-in-Publication Data
Ozonoff, Sally.
    [A parent's guide to Asperger syndrome and high-functioning autism.]
    A parent's guide to high-functioning autism spectrum disorder : how to meet
the challenges and help your child thrive / Sally Ozonoff, Geraldine Dawson,
James C. McPartland. — Second edition.
        pages cm
    Includes bibliographical references and index.
    ISBN 978-1-4625-1747-3 (paperback) — ISBN 978-1-4625-1795-4 (hardcover)
    1. Asperger's syndrome—Popular works.   2. Autism spectrum
disorders—Popular works.   3. Parents of autistic children.   I. Dawson,
Geraldine.   II. McPartland, James C.   III. Title.
    RJ506.A9O98 2015
    618.92′858832—dc23
                                                                2014026326

To Martha and Doug, who have given me
a new window on parents' experiences
—S. O.

To my husband, Joseph,
and daughter, Margaret
—G. D.

To my parents and greatest mentors,
Rosemary and Jim McPartland
—J. C. M.

Contents

Contents

Acknowledgments

The writing of this book would not have been possible without the parents and children who shared their stories, pain, hopes, and triumphs with me. I have learned far more from them than I have been able to give back. Thank you for letting me be a part of your lives at your bleakest moments and at your times of joy. I have learned so much from my mentors, Bruce Pennington, who taught me the science of autism; Sally Rogers, who taught me the art of autism; and Gary Mesibov, who immersed me in the culture of autism. Kitty Moore and Christine Benton of The Guilford Press helped greatly in the writing of this book and often knew what I wanted to say better than I did. I also thank my father, who instilled in me a love of writing and editing; my mother and my husband, who provide support and encouragement every day; my daughters, Grace and Claire, who have grown up alongside autism spectrum disorder and become experts themselves; and Jesse, who has taught us all about autism in the family and what it is really like.

—S. O.

I wish to gratefully acknowledge all I have learned from the children and adults with autism spectrum disorder and their families.

Their experiences, feedback, and creative ideas have greatly influenced my thinking and practice over the years, and their perseverance, passion, and resilience are a constant source of inspiration for me. My colleagues and students at the University of Washington Autism Center were also instrumental in the writing of the first edition of this book, especially Felice Orlich, Kimberly Ryan, and Cathy Brock. I have very much enjoyed working with the staff at The Guilford Press, especially Seymour Weingarten, Kitty Moore, and Christine Benton; this book has very much benefited from their guidance and expertise. Finally, I wish to express heartfelt appreciation for the unwavering love and support I receive from my husband, Joseph, and my children, Chris and Maggie. Without their support, my work would not be possible.

—G. D.

I feel fortunate to have interacted with so many devoted parents and wonderful people with autism spectrum disorder. My contributions to this text represent the synthesis of the lessons I have learned from you, and I thank you for working with me. It has been enjoyable to collaborate with my coauthors on this project, as well as the staff at The Guilford Press. I am grateful to those who have taught me about autism, most notably Geraldine Dawson, Felice Orlich, Julie Osterling, Ami Klin, and Fred Volkmar. The support of the team at the Yale Developmental Disabilities Clinic and the McPartland lab, especially Rachael Tillman and Emily Levy, has been crucial to this book. Thank you to my family, Tara, Norah, and Aggie, for believing in me and my work.

—J. C. M.

Authors' Note

To protect the privacy of the families we have worked with over the years, the children and parents depicted in this book for illustrative purposes are either composites of those we have worked with and represent typical situations, challenges, and solutions, or thoroughly disguised individuals.

For ease of reading, we have alternated between masculine and feminine pronouns. Unless specifically noted otherwise, statements using singular personal pronouns apply to both boys and girls (or men and women).

This book is not intended to substitute for a qualified professional evaluation, diagnosis, or treatment. Throughout the book we offer advice for finding qualified clinicians, and the Resources list medical centers and clinics that offer help with autism spectrum disorder.

Part I

UNDERSTANDING HIGH-FUNCTIONING AUTISM SPECTRUM DISORDER

1

What Is High-Functioning Autism Spectrum Disorder?

Joseph had always seemed like a brilliant child. He began talking before his first birthday, much earlier than his older sister and brother. He expressed himself in an adult way and was always very polite. When his mother offered to buy him a treat at the movies, for example, Joseph said, "No, thank you, M&M's are not my preferred mode of snacking." He showed a very early interest in letters and by 18 months could recite the whole alphabet. He taught himself to read before his third birthday. Joseph wasn't much interested in typical toys, like balls and bicycles, preferring instead what his proud parents considered "grown-up" pursuits, like geography and science. Starting at age 2, he spent many hours lying on the living-room floor, looking at maps in the family's world atlas. By age 5, he could name anywhere in the world from a description of its geographical location ("What is the northern-most coastal city in Brazil?"). Just as his parents suspected, Joseph *is* brilliant. He also has autism spectrum disorder.

Nine-year-old Seth was playing video games in the family room while his mother bustled about the house cleaning up for the guests who would soon arrive. As she climbed a stepladder in the living room to change a light bulb, she lost her balance and fell backward. While she lay on the floor gasping for breath, Seth walked by on his way to the kitchen for a snack, stepped over her, and said "Hi, Mom." Seth has autism spectrum disorder.

Clint turns 30 soon. He graduated from college with a degree in engineering, lives in an apartment in a nice section of town, recently bought a used car, and enjoys going to the movies. He is troubled, however, by his difficulty finding and keeping a job. Time and again, supervisors have gotten frustrated by his slower work pace and difficulty getting along with coworkers. Clint gets stuck on details and finds it hard to set goals that eventually lead to completion of his projects. After finishing a seasonal job cleaning hotel rooms at a ski resort, he tells prospective employers that he was "let go" without realizing that this term means "fired" to most people. Unable to find work for months, he visits a vocational counselor, who suggests a psychological evaluation. Testing reveals that Clint has autism spectrum disorder, which was never diagnosed.

Lauren is a teenager with the looks of a model. Despite her beauty, she has no friends, nor does she seem particularly interested in having any. She still loves Barbie dolls at age 17 and collects every new model and outfit that comes on the market. At school, Lauren often appears to be daydreaming; when the teacher presents directions to the class, she does not respond as she sits smiling and occasionally talking softly to herself. Despite this apparent inattention, she is a straight-A student who excels in mathematics and physics. When other kids greet her in the hallways, she sometimes does not notice and other times looks away while mumbling a quick "Hi." Now the school psychologist has mentioned to Lauren's parents that she may have autism spectrum disorder.

Joseph, Seth, Clint, and Lauren all have what is referred to as *autism spectrum disorder* or ASD. If your child resembles them in any way, you may also have heard the labels "high-functioning autism," "Asperger syndrome," or "pervasive developmental disorder" (often abbreviated as PDD). And you probably have many questions: What is ASD? What causes ASD? How is it that my unique and interesting child, who has so many strengths, could also have such challenges? What will the future bring for my child and us? This book will answer these questions and many more.

In this chapter we define some important terms to help you decide whether this book is relevant to you and whether it may help the person in your life who has similar strengths and similar challenges. We'll also tell you what we know about who has these disorders and what the future may bring to these children and their families.

The word *autism* was coined from the Greek word *autos,* meaning "self." The term was first used to describe a specific set of behaviors in 1943 by Leo Kanner, a child psychiatrist at Johns Hopkins University in Baltimore. In his landmark paper, Dr. Kanner described 11 children who showed little interest in other people, insisted on routines, and displayed unusual body movements, like flapping their hands. Many of the children could talk: some could name things in their environment, others could count or say the alphabet, still others could recite whole books, word for word, from memory. However, they rarely used their speech to communicate with others. The children had a variety of learning problems in addition to their unusual behaviors.

For many years after Dr. Kanner's initial description, only those children whose behaviors were very similar in type and severity to those of the original cases were diagnosed with autism. Slowly, however, we began to recognize that autism has a wide variety of faces and can be found in children with good communication skills, who are of normal intelligence, who have few learning problems, and who show milder versions of the behaviors Dr. Kanner described. These are so-called *high-functioning* individuals; this term has been defined in different ways but generally means having normal intelligence and a fairly good command of language. We now know that autism is not a narrowly defined condi-

5

tion, but rather a spectrum that varies in severity from the classic picture described by Leo Kanner to milder variants associated with good language and cognitive (thinking) skills. For this reason, we now use the term *autism spectrum disorder* (or *ASD*). The subject of this book is the high-functioning end of the spectrum.

Good language and cognitive skills mean that many children with ASD, like Joseph and Lauren, often do just fine in school and tend to get along well with adults. But in other ways, Joseph's unusual behaviors make life challenging. Joseph's intense interests often disrupt family activities; his parents are often unable to persuade him to leave his science projects to use the bathroom or come to the dinner table. On a recent trip to Disneyland, he insisted on taking along his globe, which had to be transported in a baby stroller throughout the park. Joseph's professor-like speech makes him stand out among his peers, who delight in teasing him and rarely accept his invitations to come over and play. Joseph has begun to make negative comments about himself ("Nobody likes me"), and his parents worry about depression. Lauren, on the other hand, doesn't seem to mind being virtually friendless, but her parents are worried about her social isolation and the social life that she is missing. A boy invited her to the junior prom, and her mother bought her a dress, but Lauren refused to go; her mother spent prom evening worrying whether her daughter would ever make any friends. Clint certainly has the intelligence to be successful, but his social awkwardness and blunt comments to coworkers ("It's too bad you broke up with your boyfriend, but we're here to work, not talk") mean that he has never kept a job for longer than a few weeks. He is also underemployed: despite a degree in engineering, Clint has held a variety of manual labor and store clerk positions. And Seth illustrates another problem that some people with high-functioning ASD have: difficulty reading other people's emotions and thus understanding empathy. Until her son was diagnosed with ASD, Seth's mother was convinced that it was something she did that had led to her son's difficulty with responding appropriately to others and their feelings. When he was young,

Seth would talk so loudly and behave so unusually in restaurants (for example, by taking food that appealed to him off other diners' plates) that the family was sometimes asked to leave. Seth's mother remembered sympathizing with a neighbor whose daughter was in a wheelchair about the restrictions their children placed on their families. The neighbor listed several things her family couldn't do, such as go hiking together, and then asked in astonishment, "What can't *you* do?" And Seth's mother, taken aback, said, "Why, we can't do anything! Seth's behavior is so active and difficult in public, but he seems so normal, that everyone gives us terrible looks. It's just too hard on us, especially Seth's siblings." These conditions can be stressful not only for the individuals who have them, but also for their families.

At about the same time that scientists began to realize that autism was a spectrum disorder and that there were high-functioning forms of it, Dr. Lorna Wing, an eminent British researcher at the Institute of Psychiatry in London, brought something called Asperger syndrome to the attention of the English-speaking world. Dr. Hans Asperger, an Austrian pediatrician, had first described children with the condition in 1944, apparently without any knowledge of Leo Kanner's work. Because Asperger's paper was written in German and published during World War II, it was not widely read. Until Dr. Wing's paper was published in 1981, the condition remained virtually unknown in the United States and other non-German-speaking countries. In her paper, Dr. Wing summarized Asperger's original publication, but she also noted the similarities between Asperger syndrome and autism, raising for the first time a question that is still with us today: Are Asperger syndrome and high-functioning autism the same disorder or two separate ones?

Asperger syndrome was first included in the manual used by doctors to make psychiatric diagnoses, the *Diagnostic and Statistical Manual of Mental Disorders* (or DSM), in 1994. People began being diagnosed with Asperger syndrome shortly afterward, and it rapidly became a popular diagnosis to describe individuals with milder forms of ASD, who had good language and cognitive skills. The question of whether it was different from autism remained, and many researchers conducted studies to try to answer this question. Over the next 20 years, dozens of investigations were carried out and research evidence accrued that, in fact, there were virtually no reliable differences between Asperger syndrome and high-functioning autism. People with the syndromes share the same challenges and the same strengths in their learning profile. They require the same treatments, respond equally well to those interventions, and have similar outcomes later in life. Their brains look similar in brain-imaging studies. And perhaps most telling, Asperger syndrome and autism seem to have the same causes. It is common for families who have two children on the spectrum to have one with Asperger syndrome and one with autism. Even within identical twin pairs, who share the exact same genetic profile, one can be diagnosed with Asperger syndrome and the other one with autism. It began to look more and more to both researchers and clinicians like high-functioning autism and Asperger syndrome were two names for the same condition. Therefore, when the diagnostic manual used by all psychiatrists and psychologists to make clinical diagnoses was revised in 2013 (abbreviated as DSM-5), Asperger syndrome and high-functioning autism were wrapped up into a single diagnosis called autism spectrum disorder (ASD). Children who would previously have met criteria for either Asperger syndrome or high-functioning autism will now meet criteria for ASD. Chapter 2 goes into more detail on diagnostic procedures, recent changes in the newest version of the DSM, and how they may affect your child and you. What is important for parents to know is that whatever the conditions are called (high-functioning autism, Asperger syndrome, ASD, or the broader term *pervasive developmental disorder*, or PDD), they present many of the same strengths and challenges and similar treatments will help individuals who have been given any of these diagnoses. The practical guidance in this book will help those with any of these diagnoses. We will use the term *high-functioning autism spectrum disorder*, or simply ASD, throughout this book to include *all* conditions.

What Does High-Functioning Autism Spectrum Disorder Look Like?

No one will display all the features that characterize ASD; some individuals will exhibit fewer features than others. Just as no two people without ASD, even identical twins, are absolutely alike, no two individuals with ASD behave in exactly the same way. All, however, have some difficulties socially interacting and communicating with other people and show some odd or repetitive behaviors.

Problems with Social Interaction and Communication

The core feature of ASD is difficulty with socially interacting and communicating with others. Challenges in this area span a wide range. The striking social impairments of more classic autism, such as social remoteness and avoidance of other people, rarely appear in higher-functioning children like those we focus on in this book, but difficulties nonetheless exist. Some children, like Lauren, don't go out of their way to start conversations or interact with others but do respond if other people approach them. Other individuals show interest in people and enjoy their company; they may even want to join groups and make friends. However, their ability to do so successfully is limited by their difficulty knowing what to do or say in social situations. They may be awkward and unsure during interactions. They may give the impression that they are not interested in the person they are talking to because they don't follow the "rules" of social interaction. Most of us naturally know that we should look at the person we're talking to, smile, and nod occasionally to signify that we are paying attention. People with ASD, however, don't seem to appreciate these unwritten rules of social engagement. Their behavior while out in public may sometimes be inappropriate or embarrassing when, in addition to failing to use these social niceties, they violate clear social conventions, such as refraining from asking overly personal questions or keeping certain opinions to themselves. It may indeed be true that your neighbor's upper arms look like "fat sausages," but this is information best kept to yourself.

People with ASD often appear not to understand other people's feelings or points of view, which makes their social interactions even more difficult. Often these abilities, natural to the rest of us, are delayed or do not develop fully even as the child gets older. Empathy usually begins emerging in infancy, when young children start to show an interest in and a concern about the feelings of others. It's not uncommon in day care centers to see babies break into sympathetic wails when another infant cries or to see toddlers take a toy or an adult to a crying child in an attempt to comfort their peer. Preschoolers are fascinated by the moods of others and often talk about friends being angry or sad. In their pretend play, young children enact scenes in which characters are sick or upset, grappling with understanding such states and how to respond to them.

In contrast, many children with ASD have basic difficulty appreciating the emotions of others (and often their own as well). As Seth's mother could attest, some, but not all, children with ASD don't notice when parents, siblings, or other children are hurt, sick, or sad, and even when they do they rarely offer comfort. Or they may horribly misunderstand others' feelings. One boy burst into laughter after his father fell down the stairs, tearing ligaments in his ankle. When his horrified mother asked why he was laughing, he explained, "Dad is jumping around and making funny faces like a clown." Clint described an interaction with a coworker who made "a strange face" after he told a joke. He didn't think much about it until later, when he saw a photograph of a woman bearing the exact same facial expression. He showed the picture to his mother and asked how the woman felt. She said, "Offended, I think." Clint has felt bad about insulting his coworker ever since, but says, "If someone is insinuating something through their face or body, without being direct, I just can't grasp it."

While most children with ASD establish warm, loving relationships and secure bonds with parents, siblings, and understanding adults, most, if not all, individuals with ASD experience difficulty relating to peers of approximately the same age. Some children are teased or bullied, others are ignored by kids, and still others, like Lauren, seem perfectly content to have no friends. Some develop friendships that revolve around shared interests (such as video games). Many children with ASD report feeling lonely and socially isolated because of such peer difficulties. They are hurt by teasing and often unaware of their unusual behavior or social responses that may contribute to the situation. In later childhood or adolescence, they can become painfully aware of their differences from others and their inability to understand the fundamentals of interaction that others accomplish naturally. One teen stated, "I know I'm supposed to look people in the eye— my parents are constantly reminding me—but it doesn't help me understand them, so I just don't do it." This can lead to low self-esteem and low self-confidence that, in a vicious cycle, perpetuate the problems. As the child loses hope of social success, he or she gives up trying to interact with others. This only increases social isolation, which may further compound the awkwardness or outright oddity of the child's social behavior. In the most extreme cases, the cycle may lead to serious bouts of depression that require treatment. Fortunately, as we will discuss later in the book, children with ASD are capable of learning how to interact socially and even interpret other people's emotions. With "social skills training," most if not all children make significant improvements, and many go on to have rewarding and successful relationships with their peers and others.

ASD also involves communication problems. A prominent feature of classic autism, at least in the minds of many people, is an inability to talk or very significant delays in speech. What is less well appreciated is that even high-functioning individuals on the autism spectrum experience difficulties with communication. This, it turns out, is one of the most confusing parts of the diagnostic puzzle and often leads to misdiagnosis when the child is young. You may have had autism raised as a possibility at some point in your child's life, only to have it "ruled out" or to be told later that he or she couldn't possibly have autism because the child speaks so well. It is now clear, however, that some children on the spectrum have very good language skills. Some children show initial speech delays and begin talking late, but soon catch up and speak fluently and articulately later on. A smaller, but not insignificant, number of children develop speech on time or even early and parents may first believe their child is gifted based on precocious language skills. Yet there are virtually always differences in the *way* language is used, particularly in social contexts, that can cause problems. The child, adolescent, or adult with ASD may dominate conversations, talking on and on without giving others the chance to say anything. The pedantic or overly formal manner of speaking that Joseph uses is common. At age 7, Joseph begins many statements the way a professor might, saying, "Actually . . ." or "I do believe. . . ." He has a vast vocabulary and loves to use unusual words—the bigger the better. When asked his favorite color, he pointed to a yellow balloon and said with a smile "chartreuse." Clint defines terms that don't need defining. He readily tells people that he is autistic, hastening to add, "*Autistic* is the adjective for the noun *autism*" as if we would not know what the word meant without this explanation. While there is nothing technically wrong with phrasing things so formally, it certainly makes Clint and Joseph stand out from their peers and often makes them the target of teasing. Joseph's mother likens his speech patterns to someone who speaks English as a second language: other people can figure out what he is trying to say, but the way he phrases even simple statements makes it seem as if English is not his native tongue.

Another communication challenge for children with ASD is their *literal interpretation* of what is said. As we all know, often what we say is not exactly what we mean. When his mother sarcastically commented that Seth, who had ignored her request to clean his room, "was doing a really good job," he nodded and continued playing video games. He didn't appreciate his mother's frustration, conveyed by her tone of voice and facial expression, or notice the mismatch between her statement and the context. Another boy, when someone called his house and asked if his mother was home, answered "Yes" and then hung up the phone. He took the question literally, rather than understanding it as a polite but indirect way of asking to speak to his mother.

Still another common communication difference shown by people with ASD is *how* they speak. Children with these disorders may speak very loudly or, conversely, too softly to be heard well. Words may tumble out of their mouths at breakneck speed or crawl out as if on a recording played at the wrong speed. Or their speech may have an unusual rhythm, with emphasis placed on the wrong words in sentences, a rising conclusion to a statement, making it sound like a question, or little inflection, giving their voice a flat tone. There may be fewer of the natural pauses we usually make in conversation, resulting in run-on speech. Or they may take breaths at unusual points during speaking, such as in the middle of a word or phrase. Often children with ASD are unaware of how different from others they sound. Like social challenges, communication challenges can be addressed with interventions that focus on conversational skills.

Unusual Interests and Repetitive or Ritualized Behaviors

The second area in which high-functioning people on the autism spectrum differ is in terms of their repetitive or ritualized behavior. You will probably have noticed that your child's range of activities is relatively focused and that he can do the same thing over and over again without getting bored. He may have very specific interests that verge on obsessions. These kids have the favorite pastimes that many children have—computers, video games, dinosaurs, astronomy—but pursue them to the exclusion of almost everything else. Many parents report that their child will stay at the computer for hours, not breaking to go to the toilet, to eat, or to sleep unless pressured, and even then with much resistance. The intensity of the child's interests seems odd to others and may contribute to the child's social isolation. So does the child's choice of interests. Few children (or adults) not on the autism spectrum appreciate the intricacies of the stock market, astronomy, sprinkler systems, or botanical classification, but these are the types of things that children with ASD tend to favor. Their interests often revolve around topics about which the child can amass a great deal of facts and information. Sometimes these children also form unusual collections. One teenage girl with ASD saved the little sticker from every banana and apple she had ever eaten, keeping them in a treasured scrapbook that she carried with her everywhere.

What many onlookers find even more puzzling about children with ASD is that, despite all the time they spend on these interests, they often do not have good commonsense knowledge of their favorite subjects. They zero in on the details but are often unable to see "the big picture." One young man with ASD was very interested in vacuum cleaners. He knew everything there was to know about vacuums: the cost, color, repair record, and number and kinds of attachments for every brand on the market. He correctly identified my (S. O.) home vacuum as "tan with chocolate-brown trim" with two attachments, one hose-like and one with a brush. Its repair record was not good, he explained to me, since most of the internal parts were made of plastic rather than metal (in fact, it did not seem to work too well!). But when asked for advice about replacing it with a better one, the boy became agitated and eventually advised me to purchase a Royal, justifying this choice by explaining that it has a blue bag. Like many individuals with ASD, he seemed unable to distinguish important details from irrelevant ones and to weigh the multiple details he had memorized. If your child has ASD, you may notice that she has the same problem with thinking in general, demonstrating an excellent memory for facts but more difficulty understanding abstract concepts and using common sense. If you give your child a rule, she may have trouble generalizing it to a slightly different situation. Your child may want to solve problems the exact same way each time and may get very frustrated when you try to help her see new solutions or ways of doing things. The difficulty with seeing relationships among pieces of information, identifying central patterns or themes, and figuring out what things *mean* can make learning challenging for children with ASD, as we discuss in Chapter 7.

Many children with ASD not only engage in repetitive behavior but also use repetitive language. For example, some children memorize things that other people say (or phrases or dialogue from videos and books) and then incorporate them into their own speech. This memorized speech is called *delayed echolalia* and, while idiosyncratic, does indicate that the child has a well-developed verbal memory. Sometimes the echoed phrases are used in an appropriate context and make sense, as when Joseph exclaimed, "Oh no, it's my worst nightmare!" (dialogue from a Disney movie) after spilling milk on one of his treasured maps. Other times the link between the phrase and the context is less clear. Seth's mother reported that as a small child he would say "He's a happy man right there" whenever he put on or took off a hat. For years, she and Seth's dad had no idea where this comment came from or what it meant. Then one day they happened to be watching an old golf video they had taped several years earlier. They were astounded to see one of the golfers make a hole-in-one and then tip his cap to the audience as the announcer said, "He's a happy man right there." Seth had associated this phrase with hats, and the two remained linked in his mind, although the phrase made little sense to others and didn't help him communicate his wants or needs.

The Strengths That Accompany the Challenges

Having ASD comes with challenges but also many strengths. In this book, we focus on both aspects of ASD and help parents learn how to minimize the challenges while capitalizing on their child's strengths. In this way, people with ASD can become happy, successful members of society who have rewarding and meaningful lives. ASD is associated with many special gifts, talents, and inclinations that come along with the challenges and make your child a very special, unique, and interesting person. Many children and teens with ASD have excellent memories. They remember details of family trips, routes around their city, or spelling lists effortlessly. Many also excel in reading. Like Joseph, they may teach themselves to read at an early age and later be able to read words aloud and spell well above grade level. Others are very advanced in visual–spatial skills, putting together complex jigsaw puzzles, reading maps, or working electronic equipment far better than their peers. We will describe ways to apply your child's special interests to the "real world," so that his incredible abilities to focus, memorize, and spend long hours immersed in a topic become invaluable strengths. You may have heard of Dr. Temple Grandin, a professor of animal science at Colorado State University, who has ASD. She combined a strong interest in animals with her visual–spatial strengths to revolutionize the design of animal slaughterhouses, making them more humane as well as more efficient. She has become an international expert on the topic, giving lectures around the world. For careers that rely on detail orientation, such as library administration, engineering, or computer science, having ASD might be an asset. Your child thinks, views the world, processes information, and has a personality style that is different but not inferior. Great strengths come with the challenges. *Our* challenge is to harness those strengths and use them to overcome the hurdles that stand in the way. Chapter 5 offers practical suggestions for meeting that challenge.

What Lies Ahead?

The combination of challenges and talents seen in children with ASD strikes fear in the hearts of many parents. Which will prevail, the child's deficiencies or the child's strengths? What can you do to make sure that your child doesn't slip through the cracks because her needs are not as extreme as those of children with more severe autism? What are your child's chances of going to college, getting a good job, and marrying? When a child displays such a mixture of challenges and strengths, it is often difficult to predict what the future holds. Of course, what may lie ahead is one of the first questions parents ask.

We see tremendous variability in individuals with ASD as they get older. Some go to college, develop successful careers, and form lasting friendships, while others continue to live with family members and are underemployed in jobs that do not take advantage of their intelligence and special abilities. Adults with ASD, such as Temple Grandin and Liane Willey, have written books that eloquently describe overcoming early challenges and successfully adapting to society (see the Resources at the back of the book). Many adults continue to have a variety of residual social and communication difficulties, however, and the rates of independent living and full-time, unsupported employment are lower than we would like to see.

Our ability to predict the future for children with ASD is still limited. While we are beginning to understand the wide range of possibilities, we don't yet know how to match specific early characteristics with later outcomes. Previous research is not as helpful as we might hope because the study participants were either diagnosed with more classic autism in childhood or diagnosed late in life (since the field did not generally appreciate the existence of higher-functioning forms of ASD until recently), and therefore did not receive the treatments that we now believe are very helpful. Dr. Kanner predicted that the outcome for people with autism might improve in the future as the disorder became better recognized and new treatments were developed—just as we've seen with bipolar disorder and other conditions that once came with a poor prognosis. Recent studies have in fact found that very poor outcomes, such as institutionalization, are rare nowadays. As individuals with ASD are diagnosed earlier and provided with state-of-the-art treatments, we expect that the rate of the best outcomes, including satisfying careers and independent living, will continue to increase. In this section, we briefly describe what is currently known about how ASD unfolds and what might happen in adulthood. Much more on this topic appears in Chapter 9.

As with many conditions that begin in childhood, both the challenges and the triumphs of ASD change over the person's lifespan. Symptoms begin in infancy, increase for a few years, usually peak in the preschool period, and then begin to level off in the school-age years. Virtually everyone with ASD improves with time and age. Children learn to express themselves through language and understand language better as time goes on. They become more and more interested in social contact, and they gain skills such as making conversation and using eye contact appropriately. Still, most children will continue to qualify for a diagnosis of ASD as teenagers and adults. A recent review investigated how often individuals "recovered" from ASD (that is, met criteria for an ASD diagnosis at one point in their lives but lost the diagnosis as they got older). Looking across many different studies, they reported that between 3 and 25% of children lost their diagnosis and entered the normal range of cognitive, adaptive, and social skills as they got older. While most individuals continued to meet criteria for ASD, many made significant improvements in social behavior and communication skills over time. However, many adults with high-functioning ASD admit they still feel somewhat awkward or unsure of themselves when talking to and interacting with others; their speech is still often very formal; and they still have trouble knowing how much to say or when to stop talking. Dr. Patricia Howlin, a psychologist in the United Kingdom who has written a great deal about outcome in adult life for individuals with ASD, concludes that while some individuals may succeed as adults, such achievements depend on the available support systems (parents, intervention programs, educational accommodations) as well as on the individual's personal characteristics and abilities. She describes how the pressure to fit into a culture with very different values can come at a high cost, including stress, anxiety, and depression. Even when adults with ASD achieve important milestones, like graduating from college and establishing careers, they sometimes struggle with independent living. Seth's mother summarized both her hopes and her fears by saying, "I bet he'll become an astrophysicist, but I might have to dress him and drive him to work."

Finding Social Support for Yourself

As you search for answers about how and why your child is so different, you may feel alone. You may have spent years feeling that no one else has a child just like yours. In fact you might never have heard of ASD before your doctor or someone else raised the issue. Actually, you're not nearly as alone as you may now feel. The most recent prevalence estimates released by the Centers for Disease Control and Prevention (CDC) in 2014 found that one in 68 children in the United States (or 1.5% of the population) are diagnosed with ASD. These numbers have been rising over the last several decades. Thirty years ago, we estimated only two to four of every 10,000 individuals had an autism-related condition, and even 10 years ago the published rate was one in 250.

Only about a third of the individuals with ASD in the CDC's 2014 study had the kinds of intellectual and learning impairments of classic autism. Fully two-thirds of the children were on the high-functioning end of the autism spectrum, without intellectual disabilities. This suggests that children like yours are actually more common than children with classic autism.

If we now think that ASD is much more common than we did a decade or two ago, a question naturally arises: Is autism increasing in frequency? Is it truly more common than it used to be, or do the rising prevalence figures simply reflect better diagnostic practices and increased awareness of the milder end of the continuum? The jury is still out. There is no doubt that diagnostic criteria have changed over the years to include milder forms of ASD and that professionals are more aware of and better trained to make accurate diagnoses, all of which would contribute to increased prevalence rates. Another influential factor in the rise of prevalence rates is the improvement in services for ASD that has occurred in the United States and other parts of the world over the last three decades. This is important because prevalence rates are calculated using records from service agencies. Very few prevalence studies go directly into communities and assess all the children to figure out how many of them have ASD. Usually, prevalence studies (like those done by the CDC) review the records of schools and community agencies that serve individuals with ASD. Therefore, if we are doing a better job of providing treatments to children with ASD, then more of them will have records in these service agencies to be counted—and prevalence rates will rise. In addition to these explanations, some scientists also suspect that environmental factors increase the risk for ASD and contribute to increased prevalence rates. This is an active area of investigation at research centers around the world. We talk more about these studies and their findings in Chapter 3.

All autism spectrum disorders are much more common in males than in females; this was recognized by both Leo Kanner and Hans Asperger and has been validated by numerous studies since their time. The CDC's 2014 report stated that 1 in 42 boys were diagnosed with ASD (over 2%), whereas only 1 in 189 girls (or about 0.5%) were affected. Another study has shown that the recurrence rate (the likelihood that a family with one affected child will have a second one) is substantially lower for girls than for boys, with only 1 in 10 younger female siblings developing

ASD, while 1 in 4 younger male siblings is at risk. In fact, boys are at greater risk than girls for virtually all developmental, behavioral, and learning disorders.

The reason that girls are affected less often than boys is not yet clear. As you will read in Chapter 3, ASD seems to have multiple causes, and more than one factor may have to be present for the disorder to develop. It has been speculated that there is something about being a girl (perhaps a different prenatal hormonal environment or sex-related patterns of brain organization) that "protects" females from ASD and other developmental problems. With such protective factors present, the risk for developing disorders is lower in girls than boys and may require the presence of more of these causative factors.

In this first chapter, we described high-functioning ASD and how it influences the lives of affected children and their families. Our goal, at this point, is to help you decide whether the diagnosis of ASD is relevant to the person in your life you are worried about and whether this book will help you in your search for answers. The next chapter will explain how professionals currently arrive at a diagnosis, which conditions can be confused with ASD, and how recent changes in diagnostic practices may affect your child and you. The more you know about the diagnostic process, the greater power you have to ensure that your child receives the most accurate diagnosis possible.

2

The Diagnostic Process

After hearing the school psychologist's concerns about ASD, Lauren's parents began reading everything they could get their hands on about the condition. The label seemed to fit Lauren well in some ways, particularly concerning her lack of friends and trouble looking people in the eye, but other features, like overly formal language and clumsiness, just didn't sound like their daughter. The school psychologist felt pretty strongly that a diagnosis of ASD explained Lauren's challenges and would help her obtain needed services, but suggested they get a second opinion, recommending an experienced local child psychiatrist. At the request of the psychiatrist, Lauren's parents obtained copies of her medical records from their pediatrician. In a report dictated after Lauren's 3-year check-up, they read, "This young girl, born prematurely, is now thriving. She is physically well developed, alert, and happy, although she is described by her parents as quite shy and fearful. We spent some time assessing development. She played alone throughout the visit and rarely looked up at the adults. She was having difficulty focusing on tasks. . . . Lauren clearly has some interaction difficulties, though her relatedness is probably okay for her age." Lauren's parents were startled that the doctor had noted, way back then, their daughter's solitariness, and were both confused and frustrated by the conclusion. Why hadn't this been figured out sooner?

At age 2, Seth was not yet talking and seemed indifferent to his siblings and parents. When people called his name or spoke to him, he didn't appear to hear them. His parents were sure he wasn't deaf, as he would perk up whenever the automatic garage door opened, even when he was in distant parts of the house. But just to be on the safe side, Seth's parents had his hearing tested. The results were perfectly normal, but the audiologist asked them if they had ever considered autism. This diagnosis was confirmed by a child psychologist at age 3. Seth was immediately enrolled in a special education preschool for children with autism. He began talking quickly and made rapid progress in all areas, such that he was able to enter kindergarten in a regular classroom with just some minimal assistance from an aide. As he began school, his parents were told that he did not have autism, but actually something called Asperger syndrome. Several years later, a psychologist working with Seth mentioned "big changes" in the diagnostic system to his parents and said he now met criteria for ASD. Who was right and why did the labels keep changing?

There are many routes through the maze of diagnosis, some direct, others taking trips down blind alleys and leading to dead ends. In this chapter, we help you find your way by explaining the specific diagnostic criteria for ASD and related conditions. We'll tell you how a diagnostic evaluation is conducted and how diagnostic decisions about your child should be made; we will also discuss conditions sometimes confused with ASD.

The Diagnostic Bible: The DSM

The diagnostic process varies from agency to agency and from professional to professional. Some evaluations are comprehensive and lengthy, others relatively quick. Some professionals will use special tests, while others will talk with you and play with your child in a seemingly informal manner. But all will be collecting specific information about your child's early development and current strengths and weaknesses in the areas relevant to ASD. As we outlined in Chapter 1, these areas are your child's social interaction and communication skills, as well as any special interests or unusual behaviors. Once this information is collected, a decision is made about whether your child meets criteria for ASD. To do this, professionals use the American Psychiatric Association's *Diagnostic and Statistical Manual of Mental Disorders* (or DSM), which outlines the specific behaviors and problems associated with all emotional, behavioral, and mental conditions. The DSM is currently in its fifth edition, known as DSM-5, which was published in May 2013. The DSM is revised every decade or two to reflect new knowledge amassed by clinicians and researchers in mental health. If your child was diagnosed some time ago, then an earlier edition may have been used, probably the DSM-IV (the fourth edition), which came out in 1994 and was used until 2013. If you live outside the United States, the manual called the *International Classification of Diseases* (or ICD) may have been used instead.

As Seth's parents heard, major changes occurred in the way we think about and diagnose ASD between the fourth and fifth editions of the DSM. Many people were initially upset about the changes and didn't understand why they were made. Parents worried that their child would lose his diagnosis and no longer be able to access services that had been helpful. Before we tell you about the current system, DSM-5, we'll provide some information about DSM-IV and why these big changes were made, so you can understand the debate and how this might affect your child.

DSM–IV

In DSM-IV, the category that contained the autism spectrum disorders was called "pervasive developmental disorders." This umbrella term was used by the authors of the DSM to differentiate autism spectrum conditions from more specific developmental disorders, like learning disabilities. Children with pervasive developmental disorders experienced difficulty across multiple (or "pervasive") areas of development (social, communication, behavior, cognition, sometimes even motor skills). In contrast, children with specific developmental disorders, like dyslexia, had problems in only one specific area (such as reading) but functioned well in other areas, like social and motor skills.

There were five specific conditions included within the pervasive developmental disorder, or PDD, category in DSM-IV: autistic disorder, Asperger's disorder, Rett's disorder, childhood disintegrative disorder, and pervasive developmental disorder not otherwise specified (PDD-NOS). Two of the conditions, namely Rett's disorder and childhood disintegrative disorder, are always associated with significant cognitive impairment and are not considered on the high-functioning part of the autism spectrum, so we will not say more about them in this book. The other three DSM-IV conditions, autistic disorder, Asperger's disorder, and PDD-NOS, all shared difficulties with social interaction, communication, and repetitive behaviors but differed in the specific number and pattern of symptoms. Children with autistic disorder (the DSM-IV term for autism) had to demonstrate at least six difficulties (or symptoms) in social interaction, communication, and repetitive behaviors from a list of 12. "High-functioning autism" was the term used for individuals who met autistic disorder criteria and had relatively normal thinking, learning, and language skills. Children with Asperger's disorder (the DSM-IV term for Asperger syndrome) showed fewer than six symptoms and, in addition, had to have typical levels of language, not only at the time of assessment, but throughout their lives—that is, no late talkers in this category. Finally, the DSM-IV diagnosis of PDD-NOS was used for children who did not meet the full criteria for either autistic disorder or Asperger's disorder, usually because they had either too few symptoms or the wrong pattern of symptoms. For example, if a child displayed four symptoms (too few for autistic disorder) and had delayed language (ruling out Asperger's disorder), the diagnosis of PDD-NOS would have been used according to DSM-IV.

New Research Brings Major Changes to the DSM

The main reason the DSM, now in its fifth edition, keeps changing is that doctors want the diagnostic system to keep pace with the rapidly expanding knowledge that comes from ongoing scientific research. The first edition of the DSM was published in 1952 and did not include autism or anything like it; neither did the second edition, published in 1968. Children with autistic-type behaviors were labeled with "schizophrenia, childhood type," if they got a diagnosis at all. Autism was not added to the DSM until the third edition, in 1980. This was because research done in the 1970s clearly showed that autism was different from childhood schizophrenia. At the time, this rearranging of the diagnostic criteria was just as major as the current changes. But imagine if the DSM had not been revised and we were still using criteria based on science from 60 years ago—no one with ASD would even have a diagnosis! So you can see why updates to the DSM, based on new research, can be very helpful.

What were the recent scientific findings that led to DSM-5? Ever since Dr. Lorna Wing brought Asperger syndrome to the attention of the English-speaking world in the 1980s, researchers and clinicians noticed the similarities to high-functioning autism and wondered how the two conditions differed. Several differences were proposed: for example, maybe children with Asperger syndrome were clumsier than those with autism; some researchers and clinicians thought that children with Asperger syndrome were more likely to have special interests (like memorizing facts about the French Revolution) than children with autism; or maybe those with Asperger syndrome were more likely to talk in a formal way (like a "little professor") than children with high-functioning autism. Over the last two decades, dozens of studies have been conducted to examine these hypotheses, and many others, about what distinguishes autism from Asperger syndrome. These investigations found very few differences between the two conditions—or none at all. It seemed that the only distinctions between high-functioning autism and Asperger syndrome were the number of symptoms (more or fewer than six) and language development at ages 2 and 3 (delayed or not). Most professionals would agree that these are small differences. Observing a group of teenagers, some of whom were diagnosed with Asperger syndrome and others of whom were diagnosed with high-functioning autism, both parents and professionals were hard-pressed to know which child had which condition. This led to a very common but unfortunate experience for many families, who received different diagnostic opinions from different doctors, with one professional diagnosing their child with Asperger syndrome and another telling them that it was actually high-functioning autism (or, like Seth, changing from one diagnosis to the other as the child got older).

An eye-opening study conducted in 2012 by Dr. Catherine Lord and a group of clinical researchers from across the United States showed how differently the diagnoses of autistic disorder, Asperger's disorder, and PDD-NOS were used at different centers. At some clinics, virtually all children were diagnosed with autistic disorder and the other two labels were rarely used. At others, PDD-NOS was the most common, and at still other centers Asperger's disorder made up half of the sample. Were there really such drastically different rates of the three conditions in different parts of the country? In fact, the study showed clearly that children at the different sites were quite similar: they had similar levels of language, intelligence, and severity of autistic behaviors. So it was nothing in the children that was leading to these vastly different rates of autistic disorder, Asperger's disorder, and PDD-NOS across the country. What differed from one center to another was how the clinicians *applied* the labels, with some centers seemingly more comfortable using certain diagnoses than others. This situation probably occurred all over the world (not just at the sites participating in this study) for the 20 years that DSM-IV was in use.

Not only was this confusing for families, but also it often had negative consequences for their child's care. In some parts of the United States and other countries, individuals with Asperger diagnoses were eligible for far fewer services than individuals with autism. So, if these are one and the same condition and children with both diagnoses share the same disabilities, it is obviously very unfair to deny services to some while providing a full range of interventions to others. Professionals hope that DSM-5 will address these inequities.

DSM-5

In response to the challenges raised by new research evidence and the problems with use of the labels we just described, DSM-5 was developed. This was a 4-year process that involved scientists and clinicians from many fields, as well as advocates from parent and community organizations. This group met regularly to discuss changes suggested by new research, develop new criteria, and then examine data to see how well the new diagnostic rules worked. The work group was given the instruction to "do no harm"—for each and every change, to make sure that it would not make things worse for patients and families, such as resulting in fewer people being eligible for a diagnosis or for services. DSM-5 was published in May 2013 and is now in widespread use throughout the United States and other parts of the world. While it is still too early to know all the effects that the changes may have on children and families, there are a few published studies that suggest it is doing a good job; we'll come back to this topic later, after telling you exactly what the DSM-5 criteria are.

In DSM-5, children like yours fall into the diagnosis of autism spectrum disorder (ASD). Unlike DSM-IV, which had a category called pervasive developmental disorders and five specific diagnoses within it, DSM-5 uses a single diagnosis, ASD. DSM-IV listed 12 symptoms and required different patterns to be met for the five different PDD diagnoses; this resulted in 2,688 different ways that an individual could meet criteria! This meant that there was tremendous variability among children and it was possible for two individuals with the same diagnosis not to share a single symptom. In DSM-5, the list of symptoms has been streamlined to seven and an individual must display at least five of them to receive an ASD diagnosis. In contrast to DSM-IV, there are only six different patterns a child may show. This will make the diagnostic process much more straightforward for clinicians and will increase reliability: since there is now just a single diagnostic label, it is much more likely that a child will receive the same diagnosis from two different practitioners than it was in DSM-IV. Families will not have to face the questions that Seth's parents did, wondering why one doctor said autism and the other Asperger syndrome.

In order to meet DSM-5 criteria for ASD, a child must show difficulties in social communication and interaction, as well as restricted, repetitive behaviors. In the social domain, there are three symptoms included in DSM-5: (1) difficulty in social reciprocity, such as engaging or conversing with others or sharing their feelings; (2) difficulty using nonverbal communication, such as eye contact, facial expressions, and gestures; and (3) difficulty developing relationships appropriate for that age level. In the restricted and repetitive behaviors area, DSM-5 includes four symptoms: (1) repetitive, unusual movements, use of objects, or speech; (2) unreasonable insistence on sameness and following familiar routines; (3) interests that are narrow in focus, overly intense, and/or unusual; and (4) over- or underreactivity to sensory experiences. More detailed descriptions of these behaviors are provided in Chapter 1. Most of the symptoms are very similar to those in DSM-IV, but one new symptom was added. Sensory issues and sensitivities were not included in DSM-IV, but research studies demonstrated that they are very common in children on the spectrum, so they were added to DSM-5.

To meet criteria for ASD, your child must display at least five of the seven symptoms listed in DSM-5—all three of those in the social interaction area and at least two of the four in the restricted/repetitive behaviors area. There are many different ways that each symptom can be displayed. For example, in the area of social reciprocity, one child may have challenges in back-and-forth conversation, while another child may ignore and avoid other people; both show problems with social reciprocity, but the manifestations of this symptom are different depending upon how affected the child is. This is a new innovation of DSM-5, in which the authors made each symptom applicable to all individuals on the spectrum, from toddlers to adults, from fluently verbal to nonverbal, from mildly to severely affected. In contrast to DSM-IV, symptoms are phrased as "deficits in" rather than "lack of" a particular behavior, making them more applicable to a high-functioning child. As clinicians switched from DSM-IV to DSM-5, they have been surprised that, contrary to their expectations, it is in many cases easier for a child to meet criteria for a diagnosis, not harder.

An additional requirement for an ASD diagnosis is that symptoms must have been present in the early developmental period. No specific age of onset is given, but it is likely that most parents will be aware of at least some of these differences in their child before the age of 5. Occasionally parents may not notice problems until their child starts school, when the social demands and expectations for behavior become much higher and differences from other children become more evident. If your child fulfills these criteria (number of symptoms, pattern of symptoms across the two domains, and when differences were first apparent), then he or she will be diagnosed with ASD.

As part of the diagnostic process, your child's doctor will also specify whether he has any intellectual impairment (lowered cognitive and learning skills), language impairment, or genetic disorder (for example, Down syndrome or fragile X syndrome), along with ASD. A full diagnostic work-up will also make sure that your child doesn't have any additional diagnoses, like depression or anxiety disorder—we will offer more on this topic later in this chapter. Finally, your doctor will make a rating of how severe your child's impairment is and what level of support she needs (the ratings given are: Level 1 "requiring support," Level 2 "requiring substantial support," and Level 3 "requiring very substantial support"). Most children with higher-functioning ASD, who have fluent language and pretty typical levels of learning and thinking skills, will be at Severity Level 1 or 2. Severity levels may decrease as the child gets older. DSM-5 states very carefully that severity categories "should not be used to determine eligibility for and provision of services" (page 51).

How Will DSM-5 Affect Us?

With the introduction of DSM-5, parents have had many concerns, particularly about whether their child will still meet criteria for a diagnosis and will continue to be eligible for government-supported therapies, educational services, or insurance coverage. One very important thing for you to know is that the educational system and the medical system can be quite different in many states and countries. Regional departments of education often have their own definitions of disability and their own criteria for who is eligible for special education services that are different from the medical community, where the DSM is used. So, if you live in a region where eligibility for special education is not based on DSM criteria, your child's services at school will not be affected by the changes in the DSM.

Even if your state or country does rely on DSM criteria to make decisions about special education eligibility, your school services should not be adversely affected by the new criteria. As we mentioned earlier, the goal of the DSM-5 work group was to "do no harm." The intent of the new criteria was to identify the same individuals who had met criteria in previous DSM versions. In fact, DSM-5 includes a very specific statement that "individuals with a well-established DSM-IV diagnosis of autistic disorder, Asperger's disorder, or pervasive developmental disorder not otherwise specified should be given the diagnosis of autism spectrum disorder" (page 51). This not only implies that your child will continue to meet criteria under DSM-5 if he did under DSM-IV but also suggests that your child does not need to get rediagnosed—that the new diagnostic label of ASD will now simply be used in place of your child's old diagnostic label. So, unless your doctor or school system tells you something different, you do not need to schedule a new assessment to make sure your child still meets criteria—you can presume that he will, unless otherwise notified.

In some situations, however, a reevaluation may be necessary and a child may actually fail to meet the criteria. Why might this happen? In DSM-IV, a diagnosis of PDD-NOS required only two symptoms, one of which had to be in the social domain. There was no requirement that the child demonstrate any repetitive behaviors, while in DSM-5, a child must display at least two.

Chad was a late talker; now, at age 9, his language has improved a lot, but he still has trouble with conversations and looking people in the eye. However, he doesn't show any other clear symptoms of ASD. He has a few close friends, is highly imaginative, and has never had any unusually focused interests or other odd or repetitive behaviors.

In DSM-IV, Chad was diagnosed with PDD-NOS because he showed some difficulties associated with the autism spectrum but didn't demonstrate either the number or pattern of symptoms required for diagnoses of high-functioning autism or Asperger syndrome. These conditions required at least two deficits in reciprocal social interaction, but Chad showed only one (difficulty with eye contact). He also demonstrated a total of only three symptoms, while at least six were required for a DSM-IV autistic disorder diagnosis.

When DSM-5 was published, Chad's parents were told by a well-meaning (but mistaken) family member that they "better get him rediagnosed." They were shocked to hear that Chad did not meet criteria for ASD. The psychologist told them that there was a new diagnostic category, called social (pragmatic) communication disorder, which seemed to better explain Chad's difficulties. She explained that children with ASD are far more repetitive and stereotyped in their behavior than Chad—his challenges were in the use of language for social purposes, such as taking turns in conversation, taking the perspective of other people when talking, and understanding ambiguous language. All of these sounded very familiar to Chad's parents. In fact, it was often hard to follow him when he was trying to tell them about his day. He often wasn't clear and didn't give enough background so that they could follow what he was saying. One day, for example, he came home from school upset, saying repeatedly, "She was so mean today," without saying who "she" was. Was it his teacher? Another child in the class? The bus driver? What exactly had "she" done? His parents needed to ask a lot of questions before they could follow his story. Chad also seemed very literal to his parents. He often did not get jokes or metaphors, and they had learned not to say things that they didn't really mean (as in sarcasm or irony). The psychologist mentioned that one treatment for these kinds of problems, called pragmatic language therapy, was offered by some speech–language therapists in the area and gave them several referrals.

The symptoms of social (pragmatic) communication disorder include persistent challenges in using verbal and nonverbal communication in a social context, as manifested by difficulties in all four of the following: (1) using communication for social purposes, (2) changing communication to fit the context or adapt to the needs of the partner, (3) following rules of conversation and narrative, and (4) using and understanding nonliteral language (humor, metaphors, sarcasm). As you can see, they do overlap with ASD—in fact, most children with ASD will display many of these symptoms. However, if a child meets criteria for ASD, social (pragmatic) communication disorder is ruled out. In Chad's case, if he had displayed repetitive behaviors, in addition to his social-communication problems, he would have been diagnosed with ASD instead.

Whenever a new diagnosis is incorporated into the DSM, further study is required to determine whether it is a helpful addition. When Asperger syndrome was first included in DSM-IV, it initially seemed like it would be a useful way to identify previously undiagnosed children. It was only after research accrued over two decades that the problems with the label became clear—that it wasn't really any different from autism in its symptoms, seemed to have the same causes, and needed the same treatments. Over the next decade, the same kind of research will need to be conducted on social (pragmatic) communication disorder to make sure that it is truly different from ASD in symptoms, causes, and treatments and that, as with Asperger syndrome, we aren't just using two different names for the same thing again.

DSM-5: A Helpful Revision?

It is still early to know how many children will lose their diagnosis from DSM-IV to DSM-5, but based on some early research we are hopeful that it won't be too many and that, when it does happen, children will meet criteria for other disorders that better fit their strengths, challenges, and treatment needs. Before each new version of the DSM is published, "field trials" are conducted to test how well the new criteria work when they are used in the community by local clinicians (not just by the kinds of experts who would be on the DSM work group). Different studies use different methods to test the new criteria. One of the most stringent ways to look at whether they are working as well as or better than the old criteria is for two clinicians to independently evaluate the same child, one using DSM-IV and the other using DSM-5. In a field trial, this process is repeated on many different children, with many different kinds of problems and diagnoses, at many different clinics and locations around the country, using many different clinicians. Then the field trial study calculates how often the two clinicians, using the two different versions of the DSM, agree that the child is on the autism spectrum. For example, what percentage of the children evaluated met criteria for autistic disorder, Asperger's disorder, or PDD-NOS in DSM-IV and also met criteria for ASD in DSM-5?

One large field trial was conducted prior to publication of DSM-5 using these methods. Overall, 89% of the diagnoses were in agreement across DSM-IV and DSM-5. Even more reassuring was that the number of diagnoses on the spectrum was actually higher in DSM-5 than in DSM-IV. That means that some of the disagreements between the two DSM versions came about because a child failed to meet criteria on DSM-IV but actually did meet criteria on DSM-5. This surprised many people and is good news for everyone who wants to ensure that children getting services under DSM-IV don't lose the rights to those services under DSM-5. Another recent study, done by Dr. Carla Mazefsky and her colleagues at the University of Pittsburgh, was conducted on adults with normal intelligence, a group who many people were concerned would be underdiagnosed by DSM-5. This study found that 93% of these mildly affected individuals met both DSM-IV and DSM-5 criteria.

There are other types of studies that are sometimes cited on the Internet or in the media, suggesting that DSM-5 will diagnose many fewer children than DSM-IV. None of these studies used the most stringent methods we just described for field trials, so the lower rates they found may be due to using less strict research techniques. Some people are concerned that the new criteria will be hard to use with toddlers and very young children who may be on the autism spectrum, and research teams are actively studying this question. As more time elapses since the first implementation of DSM-5, more studies will be conducted and we will have a more definite answer about how well DSM-5 is doing, but we are optimistic at this point based on the first published field trials.

As you have just read, there are many different ways that a particular symptom might be evident. This means that you may read accounts of ASD that do not sound like your child. You may know a neighborhood boy with ASD who seems quite different from your son. You may have heard that all children with ASD are unaffectionate, but your child loves hugs, kisses, and cuddles on your lap. Thus it is likely that some things about the diagnosis fit your child while others do not, as Lauren's parents experienced; this does not necessarily indicate that your child was diagnosed incorrectly. But how do you know?

Is the Diagnosis Accurate?

After reading the last few pages, you may wonder what the odds are that your child will be (or has been) diagnosed accurately. Or you may actually have gotten different labels for your child's difficulties, as Seth's and Chad's parents did, and want to know how to find out which one is right. Or perhaps you think the diagnosis you've gotten exaggerates or minimizes your child's problem. What do you do? When parents do not feel confident in the diagnosis their child has received, it is sometimes helpful to get a second or even a third opinion until what you're told makes sense in the context of how well you know your child and what you know about ASD. This is unfortunately a time-consuming and expensive process that many parents cannot afford. The following are our best, concise answers to questions that parents commonly raise about ASD diagnoses.

What If One Professional Says My Child Has ASD and Another Says He's Normal?

As we have emphasized throughout the first two chapters of this book, autistic-like behavior falls on a continuum. How often symptoms occur, how severe they are, how pervasive they are across different settings, how much they interfere with functioning, and how much distress they cause all factor into where your child falls on the spectrum and how close to what is considered "normal" he or she is. It's important to distinguish a diagnosis of ASD from the little quirks and eccentricities that we all have. Most symptoms of ASD can be found in some individuals without ASD, but usually in much milder form. You may well know someone who is obsessed with a topic—say, model trains or computers—but who in other ways seems perfectly typical and not at all autistic. A neighbor of mine (S. O.), who is absolutely normal in all other ways, checks a weather app on his phone a dozen times a day. He also enjoys keeping a list of when the sun rose and set in several cities around the world (usually places he and his wife have visited in their travels). Unlike people with ASD, however, he does not tell others about this interest and in fact was a bit embarrassed when I happened upon the list as I was looking for a pen at his house one day. Or you may know someone who seems at a loss for words and appears quite anxious in social situations. Or you may have acquaintances who ramble on in excruciating detail and never seem to get to the point. Or you may know people who are quite orderly and become anxious when plans change. A colleague of ours, who is a very friendly and social woman, likes to plan her entire day in advance. If someone calls an unplanned meeting or invites her to lunch on the spur of the moment, she becomes quite unsettled, avoids the change when possible, and otherwise complains heartily of the disruption in her day. Any of these folks could have ASD if, in addition to the one behavior described, they demonstrated other characteristic symptoms of ASD. However, each of these behavioral "quirks," when they occur in isolation and in the context of otherwise normal social relating and communication, are simply personality variants. What this means is that much of ASD is on a continuum with "normal" (we won't get into the debate about what "normal" actually means here). The behaviors of people with ASD are something that the rest of the non-ASD world might at times experience or that might feel "normal" to them. The difference, however, between someone who has ASD and someone who does not is the severity of the disturbance, in terms of both the number of autistic-like behaviors and how much these quirks interfere with functioning and daily living.

How Can We Be Sure Our Child Has ASD and Not ADHD . . . or OCD . . . or Something Else?

Estimates of the prevalence of ASD have soared during the past three decades. Although it is still unclear what has caused this rapid rise, as we discussed in Chapter 1, one factor that has certainly contributed to it is that as professionals and the general public have become more familiar with ASD, the number of children diagnosed has soared. And as the diagnosis has become more prevalent, misdiagnosis is also more likely. Sometimes a proper assessment by a specialist reveals that this diagnosis is wrong and that the child's difficulties are more in the realm of attention problems, depression, or something other than ASD.

One reason for misdiagnosis is that the symptoms of certain disorders do have some overlap, at least superficially, with the symptoms of ASD. For example, obsessive–compulsive disorder (OCD) is a condition in which people have persistent thoughts or ideas that they have trouble getting out of their heads; they also feel extremely strong urges to perform certain behaviors or rituals. They often like to have things "just so" and become anxious or upset if things are not how they are used to or how they expect. Chris, a 12-year-old with OCD, had a favorite number (4) and felt compelled to perform actions and repeat certain phrases he had heard four times. If he didn't do this, he would become extremely nervous. The only way he could make his anxiety go away would be by making a quick sweeping motion on the floor with the back of his hand. Such unusual rituals may be somewhat reminiscent of the nonfunctional rituals of the autism spectrum. Take Mark, for example, a young boy with ASD who screams and cries if his family doesn't shut the doors of the car and fasten their seatbelts in a clockwise order, beginning with the driver. He insists that everyone get out of the car and repeat the process in the "right" order—and his family is willing to do this to avoid Mark's serious distress that otherwise results. Mark's rituals don't make any sense to others and don't seem to be functional in any way, just like Chris's rituals. Both boys experience tremendous anxiety when things aren't done just the way they want. Yet one boy is diagnosed with OCD and the other with ASD. What is the difference?

The answer is deceptively simple. If the car door rituals were Mark's only problem, he might well have OCD. But in combination with a variety of other difficulties, including avoiding eye contact, talking on and on about viruses, and showing no interest in friends, ASD is a much more complete diagnosis for Mark. A label of OCD would account for Mark's problems only partially. People with OCD do not have trouble socially interacting and are able to converse with others in a very natural way. Other than their obsessions and compulsions, they display few unusual behaviors; it is *not*, for example, a feature of OCD to have special, highly focused interests (although this is widely misunderstood and probably accounts for many misdiagnoses). What distinguishes ASD from all other conditions with which it might be confused are social reciprocity deficits and unusual communication style. If the hallmark symptoms of ASD are present, then the child most likely has ASD, not OCD or another condition.

How do professionals decide whether the child *also* has OCD? Many people with OCD recognize that their behavior is unusual and experience it as intrusive and senseless. The majority of people with OCD are quite secretive about their rituals, realizing that other people would consider them bizarre. Indeed, the affected people themselves find the rituals bizarre and fervently wish they would go away. But try as they might to suppress them, they cannot stop themselves from performing the behavior. This is quite different from the experience of most children or adolescents with ASD, who usually have little insight into the unusual nature of their behavior, do not consider it odd or eccentric, and make little attempt to conceal it. But not everyone with OCD has good insight into the unusual quality of their rituals; this is especially true of children. So a second important consideration in deciding whether a child has ASD alone or both ASD and OCD is the desire to achieve simplicity in diagnosis. During training, most professionals are encouraged to use the fewest diagnoses possible for one individual. When reasonable, we try to summarize difficulties under one diagnosis rather than listing three or four separate conditions. This practice is sometimes referred to as the "law of parsimony" or "Occam's razor." William of Occam was an English philosopher of the 14th century who stated that it should be a goal of science to first attempt to explain unknown phenomena in the simplest manner. When applied to medical diagnostics, doctors often say, "When you hear hoof beats, think horses, not zebras." Following the law of parsimony, most clinicians would not diagnose ASD and OCD together unless the manifestations of both were clearly present and the difficulties could not be accounted for by just one of the conditions.

A number of other disorders intersect with ASD. In fact, OCD is not the most common misdiagnosis or partial diagnosis. Some children with ASD have received a previous diagnosis of attention-deficit/hyperactivity disorder (ADHD). The hallmarks of this condition, as you may be aware of and as the label conveys, are difficulty paying attention and controlling behavior and activity level. A child with ADHD may not seem to listen when spoken to or follow directions, may be reluctant to engage in tasks that are boring or effortful, may be distracted easily, fidget, leave his or her seat when sitting is expected, have difficulty waiting his or her turn, interrupt others, and talk excessively.

The similarities to ASD are probably immediately obvious. Many children with ASD display every one of these problems, but often for very different reasons than the child with ADHD. The child with ASD may not seem to listen and may not follow directions because of social deficits and language processing problems. He may not understand the centrality and importance of the human voice and may not orient to it naturally. Similarly, he may interrupt others, have trouble taking turns, and talk too much because of his difficulty reading social situations and knowing what is acceptable behavior in specific situations. He may be reluctant to do certain school assignments or have trouble staying seated, but not because these are inherently difficult tasks; they simply hold no interest for him. Praise from teachers or parents and high grades may not be incentives for the child with ASD, who has a vastly different motivation and reinforcement system than that of the typical child. He may be distracted, but not usually by the noises and other goings-on that distract the child with ADHD: the child with ASD is distracted by his own internal world, thoughts, and interests.

So one reason that children are often first diagnosed with ADHD, when in fact they have ASD, is that there is some overlap between the symptoms of the two conditions. A second reason is that ADHD is a common disorder, and thus clinicians are often more aware of it and better trained in its diagnosis than in diagnosis of ASD. Finally, the problems of ADHD (such as not remaining seated, not waiting turns, and not following directions) may be more bothersome to teachers and parents and thus may be brought to the attention of professionals more often than social awkwardness or highly specialized interests.

But just like a child with OCD alone, the child with ADHD alone does not have the problems with eye contact, conversation, range of interests, and imagination that the child with ASD has. The same approach should be taken to distinguish ASD from ADHD and the other conditions listed in Table 1 and to rule out any other apparently overlapping diagnosis. If the characteristic difficulties of ASD are present, then the child has ASD. The child receives multiple diagnoses only if all criteria for another condition are met and those features *cannot be accounted for by the ASD diagnosis.* In Table 1, we have listed some conditions that are confused with ASD.

The consequences of misdiagnosis can be serious. Obviously, it is important to know the true nature of your child's difficulties to understand her best, but accurate diagnosis is also critical to getting your child the most appropriate services. Certain treatments are designed specifically for ASD and offer the best possible outcome in adult life (more on this topic in Chapter 4). An accurate diagnosis is essential to obtaining such resources. The correct diagnosis will also steer you away from interventions that will do no good and that might even harm your child, such as medications with serious side effects and behavioral treatments that focus on the wrong issues or make incorrect assumptions about the reasons why your child acts in the ways she does.

Is It Possible That My Child Has Something Else in Addition to ASD?

Although we strive to achieve simplicity in diagnosis, it is not always possible or accurate to diagnose a child with ASD alone. Having multiple psychiatric conditions is called "comorbidity," which is very important to detect, because if the other problems are left untreated, they can lead to an overall worsening in your child's functioning. Research has repeatedly shown that individuals with ASD are at higher risk than other individuals for the conditions listed in Table 2, for reasons not fully understood yet. Several studies have shown that over half of children and adults with autism spectrum disorder have one or more of these comorbid conditions.

Professionals who are evaluating and treating children who may have ASD have to tread a fine line between overdiagnosing many disorders and failing to spot true comorbidity. Children with ASD often can't help in the diagnosis of a co-occurring condition because their self-awareness is limited and they have poor

TABLE 1. Possible Previous Diagnoses, Incomplete Diagnoses, or Misdiagnoses

Diagnosis	Features
Attention-deficit/ hyperactivity disorder	• Inattention • Hyperactivity • Impulsivity
Hearing impairment/ deafness	• Reduced or complete lack of ability to hear sounds of multiple frequencies
Learning disabilities	• Difficulty in reading, spelling, mathematics, or written language that is unexpected given age, education, and intelligence
Intellectual disabilities	• Intelligence scores below 70 • Slower rate of learning • Challenges performing activities of daily living independently (for example, eating, dressing, going to the toilet, communicating, working, playing) at levels expected for age
Nonverbal learning disability	• Math skills significantly below IQ • Nonverbal IQ significantly below Verbal IQ • Difficulty with spatial processes (puzzles, maps) • Poor handwriting • Poor motor skills; clumsiness
Obsessive–compulsive disorder	• Persistent, repetitive thoughts, actions, or rituals • High anxiety if not allowed to perform acts • Understanding that the behavior is senseless
Oppositional defiant disorder	• Negativistic, hostile, defiant, or disobedient behavior toward authority figures
Reactive attachment disorder	• Markedly disturbed social relatedness • History of significant abuse or neglect
Schizoid personality disorder	• Little interest in social relationships • Unemotional or few strong emotional responses
Schizophrenia or psychotic disorder	• Bizarre, fixed beliefs (delusions) • Unusual perceptual experiences (hallucinations) • Disorganized speech and behavior
Selective mutism	• Consistent failure to speak in social situations (for example, school) despite speaking in other situations (for example, home)
Social anxiety disorder (social phobia)	• Marked, persistent fear of social situations • Recognition that the fear is excessive/unreasonable
Speech–language disorders	• Failure to use pronunciation, vocabulary, or grammar (for example, tense, plurals) expected for age; shorter and less complex sentences • Difficulty understanding language and processing verbal instructions
Tourette syndrome	• Tics (sudden, rapid, recurrent movements or sounds)

TABLE 2. Other Disorders That Often Co-Occur with ASD

Diagnosis	Features
Anxiety disorders	• Excessive worry • Avoidance of certain situations or objects due to fear
Attention-deficit/ hyperactivity disorder	• Inattention • Hyperactivity • Impulsivity
Depression	• Sadness and/or irritability • Loss of interest in previously pleasurable activities • Changes in eating and sleeping patterns • Fatigue and loss of energy • Feelings of worthlessness, hopelessness • Suicidal thoughts or behavior
Tourette syndrome	• Tics (sudden, rapid, recurrent movements or sounds)

insight into their own emotions, difficulty reading their own and others' mental states, and limited ability to talk about abstract concepts. This is where parents and professionals who know the child well can step in. It may be up to you to spot and report any clear changes in behavior or thinking in your child, which indicates the possibility of comorbidity. ASD does not cause bad moods, so if your previously happy child becomes irritable or tense or otherwise different in his moods for several weeks in a row, you may want to take him to a psychiatrist or a psychologist to explore whether depression or anxiety is complicating the ASD. Similarly, if he suddenly develops a new behavior, such as deliberately injuring himself or being quite aggressive toward others, you should seriously consider a visit to your doctor to find out whether another condition may be emerging alongside the ASD. Finally, if your child does not respond to treatment interventions as you and your doctor expect, then you should examine whether there is more going on than ASD alone. You should always raise the question of comorbidity at an initial assessment if you feel that your child's behavior doesn't fit the typical ASD profile and you suspect there is more going on.

The Assessment Process

The exact sequence of events in the assessment process will vary depending on who does the evaluation and where. But let's start with the assumption that your child has been referred for an evaluation because you, a teacher, or someone else who has observed your child closely is concerned that a developmental problem may exist.

Who Is Qualified to Diagnose ASD?

The types of professionals most often making such diagnoses are psychologists, child psychiatrists, and pediatricians. Other types of doctors, such as neurologists and general practitioners (sometimes called "family practice doctors"), may also see your child for a diagnostic evaluation. Additionally, social workers are trained in the diagnostic process and how to use DSM-5, so they are qualified to make diagnoses. Other professionals, such as teachers, speech–language pathologists, and occupational therapists, may have some knowledge of ASD and may well be the ones who first alert you to the possibility, but they are usually not trained in the diagnostic process. Since teachers and therapists often have experience with other children like your son or daughter, even though they cannot make a formal diagnosis, you would be wise to listen to their concerns and ask for a referral to a qualified professional. At some agencies and clinics, your child will be seen by a team of professionals from a wide variety of disciplines, including psychology, psychiatry, pediatrics, education, social work, and speech–language therapy, so you and your child will get the benefit of even the professionals who are not, by themselves, able to make a diagnosis. At other agencies and clinics, your child may be seen by a single professional who makes the diagnosis alone; this is fine (and can be as good as a team evaluation), as long as the doctor has the appropriate expertise.

Are You Getting the Expert Help You Need for a Good Diagnosis?

Many different types of professionals are qualified to diagnose ASD. In our experience, expertise in the area of ASD is much more important to a thorough, accurate diagnosis than particular credentials. It can be difficult to know whether you have found the best person to evaluate your child, however, until you go through the process. Here are some questions to ask yourself as the evaluation proceeds. Any "no" answers should prompt you to ask the professional for an explanation, more information, or further evaluation. If you're not satisfied by the explanation, or you get a number of "no" answers, consider seeking another professional for a second opinion once the assessment is finished.

- Did the doctor interview you about your child's early history?
- Did the doctor spend at least 30 minutes with your child to observe his or her behavior?
- Did the doctor meet with you to explain the results of the assessment and answer your questions?
- Did the doctor's feedback seem to fit your child? Did the doctor understand the problems your child is experiencing that prompted you to seek the evaluation?
- Did the doctor explain which diagnosis best fits your child and why?
- Did the doctor give you options for treatment that are available in your community and specific referrals (phone numbers and the like)?
- Did the doctor provide or promise to provide a report that summarizes the results of your child's testing?

Whatever his or her particular credentials, the most important quality for your diagnostician is knowledge of and experience with ASD. It is not uncommon for professionals without such training, even those with appropriate degrees, to mistake higher-functioning ASD for something else. Just as you may have thought of a very remote, silent child obsessed with spinning objects in a corner when you first heard the term "autism," so too many professionals without appropriate training think that a verbal, bright child who does not flap his or her hands cannot possibly have anything related to autism. This is likely what delayed both Lauren's and Clint's diagnoses. So be sure to ask, when scheduling an appointment for a diagnostic evaluation, if the examiner or team has expertise, or at least experience, with higher-functioning ASD.

Developmental History

The two essential ingredients in a diagnostic evaluation are an observation of your child and a thorough parent interview, including a developmental history and questions about when your child achieved milestones like talking and walking. You, the parents, tell the professionals in detail what your child is like at home, on a day-to-day basis, since some of both her strengths and her difficulties might not be apparent during the observation period. ASD involves two different kinds of symptoms: (1) typical behaviors that fail to develop (for example, empathy, close friendships, pretend play, and eye contact) and (2) unusual behaviors that are not present in other children (for example, echoing from videos, obsessive interests, or extreme anxiety over changes in routine). The evaluator will ask you specific questions about these behaviors, both what they are like at the present time and how they were when your child was young, before age 5.

Observation of Your Child

The professional will also observe your child and interact with her for some period of time, making note of the same types of symptoms he or she asked you about in the interview. The examiner might set up specific situations to make sure that certain symptoms, if present, are evident during the observation period. Eye contact, for example, is often poor in children with ASD. To be certain that your child's eye contact is limited with the examiner because of ASD and not just due to shyness or lack of opportunity, the examiner might set up explicit scenarios that powerfully pull for eye contact, such as making it necessary that your child ask for help or doing something unexpected, such as offering a broken toy. In such situations, typical children almost always make eye contact. Similarly, the examiner might ask your child to tell a familiar story, because most typically developing children will periodically make eye contact to be sure that you are following them or are interested in what they are saying. An experienced evaluator might engineer a specific opportunity for your child to empathize with her to examine this criterion accurately. She might pretend to stub her toe or might mention that something sad happened to her recently (such as that her favorite pet was lost) to gauge your child's reaction and ability to offer comfort or support to others.

In most cases, the parent interview and direct observation of your child are enough for the examiner to make or rule out the autism spectrum diagnosis. As may already be apparent, there is no *medical* test for ASD. We cannot draw blood and look at chromosomes or levels of any particular chemicals to tell us whether your child has ASD. We can take pictures of his brain (for example, with magnetic resonance imaging [MRI] scans), but that won't tell us his diagnosis. As you will read in Chapter 3, we have found a few brain abnormalities in some people with ASD but nothing present in all (even most) people with ASD—and most of these brain differences can be found in people who don't have ASD too. Currently there are no specific biological tests for ASD. Professionals rely on the presence of the specific behaviors described in this chapter to diagnose the conditions. But this is not necessarily the problem it may sound like. All disorders in DSM-5 are diagnosed on the basis of behavior (rather than biology), and ASD happens to have among the very highest reliability of these disorders. That means that if several different professionals were to see the same child with ASD, they would be more likely to agree on his diagnosis than were they to see a child with another (less reliable) diagnosis, such as ADHD.

Medical Tests: Informative But Not Usually Diagnostic

A related question you may have is whether specific medical tests might be helpful in your child's evaluation, even though they might not be critical to making the actual diagnosis. The answer to this question varies from child to child. Some children have certain risk factors or events in their history that make a full medical work-up highly desirable. For example, approximately 25% of children with ASD also have seizures, which can range from short lapses of attention or staring spells to violent convulsions of the entire body. Seizures are most common in more severely affected children with ASD but can also occur in individuals with milder symptoms. The most common periods in which seizures start are preschool and adolescence. If your child has ever displayed behaviors indicative of potential seizures, then neurological testing, such as an electroencephalogram (EEG) and/or an MRI (brain scan), may be ordered by your doctor. If your child went through a stage of development in which he or she lost skills (for example, learning to talk and then losing the ability to speak), neurological testing may again be warranted. All children should have genetic testing, because in a minority of cases ASD is associated with identifiable genetic conditions such as fragile X syndrome. If your child has anything slightly unusual about his face, hands, feet, or skin, he should be seen by a medical doctor. For example, if he has multiple brown or white birthmarks on his skin, large or unusually shaped ears, or other minor differences in how he looks, he may have a genetic condition that underlies his autism that might require additional medical treatment and genetic counseling. If other members of your family, including your siblings, nieces, nephews, and other children, have been slow or unusual in their development, this may warrant genetic testing and genetic counseling.

Psychological Tests

Just as there are medical tests that are not diagnostic, but that are informative, so also there are behavioral or psychological tests that are not needed for the diagnosis but nevertheless can be very helpful in painting a complete picture of your child's strengths, weaknesses, treatment needs, and so forth. Probably the most common additional psychological testing that will be done during a diagnostic evaluation is an intelligence (or IQ) test.

Intelligence Tests

For verbal children over age 5, the test that is used most often is the Wechsler Intelligence Scale for Children, or WISC (pronounced "whisk"). It provides three different IQ scores, one measuring verbal intelligence, another measuring nonverbal intelligence, and a third combined score. The WISC, like the DSM, is revised periodically, both to improve its reliability and to update its norms. It is currently in its fourth edition and so is known as the WISC-IV ("whisk-four"). If your child is over age 17, he or she may have been given the adult version, the Wechsler Adult Intelligence Scale, Fourth Edition (or WAIS-IV, pronounced "wace-four"). If your child is under age 6, a variety of different tests may be used, including the Mullen Scales of Early Learning, the Stanford–Binet Intelligence Scale, the Leiter International Performance Scale, and others. If your child has taken one of these tests within a year or so, perhaps at school, the evaluator may just review the scores, rather than retesting the child now (this has an added financial advantage, as testing done through the school is free). Be sure to take any records of earlier testing to your appointment so that your doctor can use these previous scores whenever possible.

It's often useful to know the broad range in which your child's intelligence falls so you can plan the most appropriate educational interventions. It is probably a good idea, however, to view your child's IQ scores with some caution. Children with ASD often have attention and motivation problems that affect their test-taking performance and may cause them to score lower on IQ tests than their true ability. Furthermore, IQ scores reflect the "average" of all the different subtests that are given, and children with ASD often show greatly varying levels of ability across the subtests. Thus, the average score may not be that meaningful as a true reflection of your child's abilities. IQ test scores need to be interpreted in light of the child's behavior during the test itself. They may also change as your child gets older and becomes better at taking tests. And you need to know what the three different IQ scores indicate. The individual verbal and nonverbal IQ scores should not be viewed as absolute indications of your child's intellectual potential. Even the overall combined score should be considered within the broader context of your child's behavior and accomplishments in everyday living, which are also measures of intelligence. But in the case of children with ASD, IQ scores may be even less accurate than in typical children who don't have some difficulty communicating and relating to others. Due to social difficulties, for example, your child might not care about the examiner's reinforcement ("You're working hard") and thus not be motivated to perform her best on the IQ test. Or his unusual style of speaking might be an obstacle on certain tests. For example, when asked to define the word *glove*, a child with ASD might say, "a hand covering not in fashion these days unless it is a cold season" rather than give the more typical answer, "something you wear on your hands when it is cold." The first definition is not among the options for correct answers in the IQ test manual and therefore would not receive full credit. For these reasons we advise all parents, but parents of children with ASD in particular, to pay more attention to the *range* of functioning that your child's score falls into, rather than the specific number. You may be told, for example, that your child is functioning in the "average" range, the "superior" range, or the "borderline" range. The average score on all IQ tests is 100. Children obtaining scores below 70 are considered intellectually disabled. Those with scores from 70 to 80 fall in the borderline range, from 80 to

90 in the low average range, from 90 to 110 in the average range, from 110 to 120 in the high average range, from 120 to 130 in the superior range, and above 130 in the very superior range. So if your child is on the low end of the average range, he or she may well need extra help in school (more on this topic in Chapter 7). Certain IQ patterns also may indicate learning disabilities and the need for further testing.

As mentioned earlier, you will probably be given at least three IQ scores by the examiner interpreting the results. All are on the same scale just described (with an average of 100). The Verbal IQ score indicates how well your child performed on tests that require language—for example, defining words, remembering lists of numbers, and describing how two things are related. The Performance IQ score measures how well your child carries out tasks that don't require language but rely on visual–spatial skills, such as putting together puzzles, finding the way out of mazes, and putting cards in order to tell a coherent story. These two scores can be combined into a Full Scale IQ score that indicates your child's *overall* functioning across both verbal and nonverbal tasks. Sometimes your child's three scores will be similar, indicating that he or she is equally good at verbal and nonverbal tasks, but other times they can be quite different, with your child performing very highly on one kind of test but much more poorly on another kind. In such situations, the overall Full Scale score will fall somewhere in between the two extremes.

Additional Tests

Your child's evaluation may also include educational testing that examines how well he or she reads, spells, performs math calculations, writes, and so on; speech–language testing; neuropsychological testing that looks at memory, spatial processing, and the like; an occupational therapy evaluation of motor and sensory issues; and many other things, depending on how comprehensive the team conducting the evaluation is. All these areas are of some interest in that they produce the most complete picture of your child, but parents and professionals sometimes have to weigh the desire to be comprehensive with practical constraints, such as finances. If the professional is appropriately trained, a relatively quick evaluation that includes only a parent interview and an observation of your child and contains none of these "extras" can still provide an accurate diagnosis. The signs of ASD are readily discernible to the experienced professional who has asked the right questions and noticed the right aspects of behavior, without additional testing. Be sure to ask the doctor or team assessing your child how many children with ASD they see. Or call your state autism society to obtain a referral to an experienced professional. The Internet also contains websites that include lists of qualified doctors by state.

After the Diagnosis

When they first receive a diagnosis of ASD, parents experience a wide range of reactions, from one extreme of shock, grief, or denial to another extreme of relief and even happiness. More commonly, there is a mixture of negative and positive feelings. Many parents have known for a long time that there was something different about their child and have actively sought an explanation, but still hope that nothing is really wrong and their fears will prove unfounded. Parents worry about the stigma of a label, about the future, and about their child's ability to live independently and be happy. They wonder if they need to change their expectations for their child or treat the child differently. But with a diagnosis comes the promise of intervention and support. If a condition is common enough to have a name, then perhaps there is something known about how to treat it. And there must be others with this condition! You will meet other parents who know exactly what you are going through and who have great ideas about how to live with and enjoy ASD in your family. You will come to understand why your child does what she does, what motivates her, what tickles her, what is hard for her, and why. With a diagnosis comes some ability to share her perspective and see the world through the eyes of your special child. Two parents now share their stories:

"Like all parents, we had high hopes for our son, Clark. Our first two children developed fine, and naturally we assumed that Clark would follow in their footsteps. But by 18 months it was clear something was off—Clark was a happy baby, but he wasn't talking or walking, two missed milestones that are difficult to ignore. So we started down the rabbit hole of specialists. Was he hard of hearing? Did he have cerebral palsy? Was he simply a late bloomer? The initial possibilities seemed endless. But after a year and a half of searching, we finally came upon ASD. In many ways it was a relief to have a diagnosis— something to research, understand, and ultimately accept. But at the same time it was difficult to hear that your hunches were correct—not only was there something 'wrong,' but it was sad and scary and by all accounts lifelong. With time, though, we came to accept—even embrace—Clark's diagnosis. We have learned how to temper our expectations, but also to control our fears. Would he ever talk—or walk or read or make friends? The answers proved to be a resounding 'yes' to all and, although it was not the route we would have willingly taken, we are incredibly full of pride for all those milestones that took just a little longer to reach."

"Timmy turned 7 the day we received the diagnosis of ASD. Finally, the exhaustive search to discover what made our son so different—so special—had ended. A sense of relief overwhelmed us. At last we had the answer, the answer that would give purpose and direction to our long journey. Now we could focus all our efforts on learning everything possible about ASD. Now our doctors and therapists would have a unified goal. We had traveled far, but our journey had really only just begun. We felt almost joyful. The doctor thought we were crazy."

What Should I Tell My Child?

Parents often ask about sharing the news with their child. The first issue is usually "*Should* we tell him [or her]?" The answer to this question depends very much on the child's age, temperament, and other life circumstances, but usually the answer is "Yes, at some point." The next question, then, is *when?* The best way to determine whether your child is ready to hear about ASD is if he is expressing awareness of his differences, particularly voicing concerns, as when Joseph says "Nobody likes me" to his parents. Almost all the school-age children we diagnose are highly aware that they are different from others. Some are concerned, like Joseph, while others are not, but most can readily articulate that they are unlike other kids. Many children with ASD attribute this to some terrible flaw. "I have a bad brain," one boy told the first author (S. O.). After harboring hidden fears about himself for so long, finding out about ASD was a tremendous relief for this child. He heard that, yes, he is different, but his differences are very special. They include things he is really good at, as well as a few things he is not so good at but for which help is available.

This brings us to the third issue: *how* to share the news. The following is relevant for telling not only your child, but also siblings, grandparents, friends, and neighbors, about ASD (more about disclosing diagnosis in adulthood appears in Chapter 9). It is critical that the way the diagnosis is framed be positive, emphasizing your child's strengths and special skills. In discussing the difficulties that are part of ASD, we often find it helpful to compare it to a learning disability. You can ask your child whether she knows anyone who has trouble with reading, or math, or paying attention and staying seated. Emphasize that most of us have weaknesses of some sort or another; some people wear glasses, others walk with a cane, others are slow readers, others are very clumsy on the playground. But those people aren't bad at everything; there are many things they can do well. You might say, "The girl in your class who can't read well can do math just fine, has lots of friends, and is good at sports. You, with ASD, are like that too. You have trouble making friends, looking others in the eye, and knowing what to say in a conversation [choose the specific difficulties your child has that she is aware of]. But you have a great memory, you are the best speller in your class, you are good with computers, and you know so much about U.S. presidents and Brazil." Help your child understand that diversity is wonderful and that it is highly desirable to have people who are "different" among us. (There is a very helpful appendix in Liane Willey's book, *Pretending to Be Normal*, on explaining ASD to other people; choosing who, when, and how to share this news; and dealing with reactions.)

Begin the process of embracing the characteristics of ASD, for both your child and you. For this is who your child is. Take away the symptoms of ASD, and your special, much-loved child would be gone, replaced by a different child with, yes, not the same problems, but also, not the same personality, unique characteristics, and strengths. You will learn that living with ASD can have many challenges, but also great rewards that are uniquely yours to cherish.

3

Causes of Autism
Spectrum Disorders

Seth's mother had experienced an uneventful pregnancy, and Seth's delivery had been without complications. In fact, Seth's mother had no concerns about her son's development until he was about 10 months of age, when she noticed that he was not babbling like other babies of similar age. He had experienced many ear infections and chest colds as an infant and young child. His mother always wondered if this had anything to do with his ASD.

Chad had seemed like a perfectly normal baby until a few months before his second birthday, when he stopped saying the few words he had been learning and seemed to lose interest in other people. Later, his family wondered if his onset of ASD was related to the stresses associated with a family move to another home at that time. Were the two connected?

Lauren's mother had an extremely difficult pregnancy. She had high blood pressure and was placed on total bed rest for 6 weeks. Her amniotic fluid levels were low, and the baby rarely moved. Her doctor was worried about fetal distress and induced labor with Pitocin a month early. Lauren was born weighing only 5 pounds. She required resuscitation at birth and remained hospitalized, on oxygen, for 2 weeks. Could these complications really be just a coincidence, or were they related to Lauren's difficulties?

The three cases presented above make a couple of key points. First, each child with ASD has a unique developmental history, making it difficult to sort out which factors that are specific to that child's early development might have contributed to autism, if any. Second, it is natural for parents to draw connections between certain events, such as a difficult pregnancy or family move, and the cause of their child's ASD. Yet we know that other children who experience similar events don't usually develop ASD. In most cases, it is difficult, if not impossible, to identify a single factor that could explain why a child developed ASD. However, scientific research has started to provide some general answers about the causes of ASD, and we will be reviewing that knowledge in this chapter. There is clear evidence suggesting that ASD is biological in origin and not caused by parenting or other psychosocial causes related to the parent–child relationship. It is also clear that ASD does not have a single cause. Rather, ASD is a spectrum of varying severity, and different individuals will have different underlying causes for their ASD, which include a combination of genetic and environmental factors.

Brain Differences in ASD

When Dr. Kanner first described autism in 1943, he wrote that children with the disorder were born with an "innate," or inborn, difficulty bonding with people. In the mid-20th century, most doctors were trained in the psychoanalytic tradition, which attributed all behavioral and mental disorders to early childhood experiences. Thus, autism was suspected to be caused by the social environment rather than by biology. Dr. Kanner was influenced by these ideas. Later he and others blamed autism on parents. They described "refrigerator mothers" who were so emotionally cold and rejecting that they caused their children to retreat into an autistic "cocoon" of safety. This view began to lose credibility in the 1960s, however, after Dr. Bernard Rimland published *Infantile Autism: The Syndrome and Its Implications for a Neural Theory of Behavior*. In this 1964 book, the author attacked parent causation theories and pointed out that there was absolutely no research data to support them. He was the first to suggest that autism was due to differences in how the brain worked. This suggestion has stimulated a good deal of research into possible brain differences in individuals with ASD.

To understand where the information collected to date comes from, you need a rudimentary grasp of the methods used to study the brain. *Structural imaging*, such as magnetic resonance imaging (MRI), provides a picture of the brain's anatomy or structures, including the fibers that link one part of the brain to another. *Postmortem* or *autopsy studies* examine the brains of people who have died. This method permits scientists to look at the brain in a much more detailed manner. Researchers are actually able to examine individual brain cells (called neurons) rather than the large structures, composed of millions of neurons, captured by MRI. *Functional imaging*, including functional MRI (fMRI), measures how the brain *works*. By studying patterns of blood flow while a person is engaged in a task, for example, scientists can study whether the same parts of the brain are active (and working as hard and as efficiently) in individuals with ASD as they are in persons without ASD. Figure 1 illustrates some of the major structures of the brain and how they affect social behavior.

Autopsy Studies

Autopsy studies have uncovered some differences in the brains of persons with ASD. First, they have found that there are too many brain cells (neurons) in parts of the brain that support social and emotional behavior (*amygdala*) and learning (*hippocampus*).

Frontal lobe
- Social cognition
- Theory of mind

Hypothalamus
- Maternal behavior

Amygdala
- Recognition of emotional significance
- Social orienting/affiliative drive
- Emotional learning
- Arousal

Temporal lobe
- Recognition of facial expressions
- Interpretation of biological movement

Fusiform gyrus
- Face perception

FIGURE 1. Social brain system. Adapted by permission of Robert T. Schultz.

Moreover, the cells are smaller and more tightly packed together than they are supposed to be. This may mean that they do not have the correct shape and/or enough room to make the connections with other brain cells that allow them to function as they should. Autopsy investigations have also revealed significantly fewer brain cells in another part of the brain called the *cerebellum*, which is important in both motor coordination and cognitive activities. While these findings are very interesting, they are based on the study of relatively few brains (approximately 25) and were not found in all the brains examined. Thus we are not sure how widespread these brain differences are in people with ASD. Additionally, almost all the brains studied came from individuals with severe autism and intellectual disability, and in some cases epilepsy, and therefore we are not yet sure whether these results pertain to children or adolescents with milder forms of ASD.

Structural Imaging Studies

This research method has found a wide variety of differences among brains of persons with ASD as compared to those with typical development. One difference is found in the *ventricles* of the brain, which (in all people) contain fluid instead of brain tissue. Some studies have found that the ventricles are larger than normal in some people with ASD, which may mean that brain tissue around the ventricles has been lost. This finding is not specific to ASD, however; it has been found in a variety of other syndromes. It appears to be a marker for an abnormal brain, rather than unique to ASD.

Other studies have found that there are differences in the way the brain develops in children with ASD, and these differences can be seen very early in life. During the preschool years, young children with ASD usually have increased brain size, especially in the frontal and temporal lobes. These brain regions are known to be involved in social and language functions. However, this accelerated brain growth starts to level off by the early elementary school years. By adulthood, the brain size of persons with ASD does not differ from that of typical individuals. This unusual pattern of brain growth might be related to the development of the individual cells in the brain (neurons). During normal brain growth and development, there is at first a period of tremendous overproduction of neurons and the connections between neurons: the brain grows more cells and makes more connections than it really needs. Later, many of the neurons die and the connections between neurons that aren't being used much are weeded out. Some scientists believe that the large size of brains in some individuals with ASD indicates that this "pruning" mechanism has failed. This might mean that there is more background "noise" (or static) in the brain, which prevents it from functioning most efficiently. This is currently only a hypothesis, and we do not yet know what causes the brain to be larger or how this directly affects the way the brain functions in people with ASD.

A recent study suggests that differences in structural brain development can be seen even before ASD is diagnosed. By following a group of infants who were at risk for ASD (because they had older siblings with ASD), researchers found that 6- to

12-month-olds who later developed ASD themselves had atypical development of the fiber tracts that connect one part of the brain to another (also called white matter). These connections are important because complex behaviors such as social interaction and language require many different parts of the brain to work together. As the brain develops, the different parts of the brain become functionally connected through these fiber tracts. If these connections are not developing normally, this might help explain why individuals with ASD have difficulty with social and language skills.

Functional Imaging and Other Studies of How the Brain Works

Two specific areas of the brain have been the focus of investigations into whether the brains of those with ASD work differently from the brains of those without ASD.

Frontal Lobes

Since ASD always involves social deficits and repetitive behaviors, the areas of the brain that control these functions have been a focus of neuroimaging studies. In the late 1970s, two American neurologists, Drs. Antonio Damasio and Ralph Maurer, published a paper that pointed out behavioral similarities between people with autism and patients with damage to their *frontal lobes* (the region in the front of the brain, just behind our eyes and forehead). Both groups had difficulty controlling their emotions, would get very upset by small changes, were compulsive (wanting things to be "just so"), and were rigid in their solutions to problems, seeing things in a concrete, black-and-white manner. This led to a theory, still influential today, that if the frontal lobes do not develop correctly, this could cause autism. Functional imaging studies have found differences in how the frontal lobes are working in people with ASD. For example, for individuals with ASD, there is both less blood flow to and less electrical activity (firing of neurons) in this region, suggesting that their frontal lobes are not as active as they are supposed to be. In people without ASD, it is typical that multiple brain regions are needed to perform a task. Some studies of individuals with ASD have found that the activity of the frontal lobes is not well coordinated with other parts of the brain during task performance. Studies of normal volunteers and people with frontal damage have shown us that the frontal lobes are important to planning, flexibility, organization, behavioral control, and reasoning. If they are not working as efficiently or as well as they should, this could explain some symptoms of ASD.

Temporal Lobes

A second region of specific interest in ASD is the *temporal lobes*, which lie on the sides of the brain, roughly at the level of the ears. The specific part of the temporal lobes that seems to be involved is their very inner lining, lying closest to the center of the brain. This region is known as the *medial* (or middle) *temporal lobes*. Some of the structures in this area include the amygdala and the hippocampus. These parts of the brain are important for recognizing the emotional significance of a stimulus (for example, an angry face), interpreting emotions and facial expressions, such as where another person is looking, and memory. Some autopsy and structural MRI studies have shown differences in the temporal lobes (for example, being larger than normal early in life or having too many small, densely packed neurons). Several studies, including those conducted by two of us (G. D. and J. M.), have shown that individuals with ASD do in fact have problems in processing basic aspects of social information, including face recognition and discrimination of facial expressions—processing that is controlled by parts of the temporal lobes.

For example, in a study published in 1999, Dr. Simon Baron-Cohen and his colleagues measured brain function (using fMRI) while people with and without ASD looked at pictures of eyes.

Their job was to decide what emotion the eyes conveyed. These researchers found that adults without ASD relied heavily on both the amygdala and the frontal lobes to perform this task. In other words, these two regions seemed to be most important to processing the social and emotional information conveyed by the eyes. In contrast, adults with ASD used the frontal lobes much less than the normal adults and did not "turn on" the amygdala at all when looking at the pictures of eyes. Instead, they used other parts of the brain that are normally not active during this task. Another study, led by Dr. Robert Schultz at Yale University, found that people with ASD used the part of the brain that normally makes sense of objects when they looked at faces. Dawson and colleagues discovered that some very young (3- to 4-year-old) children with autism fail to show recognition of a familiar face, but show normal recognition of familiar objects. The brain systems responsible for interpreting information from others' faces come on line very early in life, offering the possibility that face-processing impairments may turn out to be one of the earliest indicators of abnormal brain development in autism. These findings don't mean that your child does not recognize you. Instead, they suggest that your child may rely more on cues other than facial features for recognition (such as touch and voice).

These findings suggest that one reason people with ASD may make less eye contact and may have so much more trouble understanding others' emotions, thoughts, and intentions is that critical regions of the brain are not working when they should be. Even when people with ASD can figure out what someone's eyes or face conveys, they do so in a different way than everyone else, which may be less efficient or take more time. Indeed, as you can see in the picture of the brain on page 60, many areas of the brain are involved in social behavior. Researchers are actively discovering which parts of this complex system do not function properly and therefore account for the difficulty that those with ASD have in relating socially.

Differences in the Connections among Brain Regions

As we mentioned earlier, structural imaging studies have found that the fiber tracts, or white matter, that connect different parts of the brain are not developing normally in persons with ASD. Studies using functional imaging have also supported the idea that ASD is associated with abnormal patterns of brain connectivity. Using fMRI, as well as measures of electrical activity in the brain, researchers have shown that, when people with ASD perform complex tasks, such as language, the different areas of the brain that are required for processing language are not functioning in a synchronized fashion. This may help to explain why it is often difficult for even high-functioning people with ASD to perform well when they are required to understand and respond to rapid and complex language and social information. Interestingly, this unusual pattern of brain connectivity might also help explain some of the special talents and strengths that many people with ASD have. These strengths often rely on the specialized expertise of one brain region, such as the ability to recall visual detail.

Summary

The field has come a long way since parents were considered to be the cause of ASD. Study after study finds brain differences in people with ASD. These differences appear very early in life and may help to explain both the difficulties associated with ASD, such as impairments in complex behaviors like social interaction, and the strengths. The sophistication of imaging tools is increasing rapidly but has likely not yet reached anything close to their eventual capacity. The techniques used a decade ago, when much of the research just reported was performed, were far less powerful and may have been able to identify only the most obvious brain differences. The next decade holds great promise for finding more answers about the brain differences in people with ASD and how they may cause the condition. In contrast, much progress has already been made in understanding how genes may contribute to the development of ASD.

Genetic Influences in ASD

In the 1970s, two eminent psychiatrists made an important discovery that opened the door to the study of genetic influences in ASD. Sir Michael Rutter is a famous British child psychiatrist who was knighted by the queen of England for his important research contributions to the understanding of ASD and other childhood disorders. Dr. Susan Folstein is a prominent child psychiatrist in the United States who has published many papers on the genetics of autism. Both scientists noted that, while the rate of autism in siblings was small, it was much, much higher than the rate in the general population. This led to the birth of a new field, the study of genetic contributions to autism. There is now very strong evidence that in most (but perhaps not all) families, genetics plays some role in the development of the condition. Unfortunately, it is already abundantly clear that untangling the genetics of autism will not be simple. We now know that hundreds of genes are involved in increasing the risk for ASD, and different families carry different sets of genes. It also appears that the genes have broader effects than just ASD itself. A variety of different conditions, such as language delay and learning disability, seem to run in the families of children with ASD that may all be caused by the same genes. Thus, ASD is just one of several possible outcomes of having these genes.

One piece of evidence that ASD has a genetic basis comes from twin studies, which have found that the likelihood that twins would both have autism was much higher if the twins are *identical*, that is, shared all their genes, than if they are *fraternal*, that is, shared on average only about half of their genes. Studies also showed that while many co-twins have full-blown ASD, others demonstrated language, cognitive, or social difficulties that fell short of an ASD diagnosis but were nevertheless significant clini-cally. Many scientists now believe that the genes involved do not cause ASD itself but instead cause a variety of language and social differences, of which ASD is the extreme form.

Some children with known genetic disorders have ASD, pro-viding another piece of evidence that ASD can have genetic ori-gins. Fragile X syndrome and tuberous sclerosis are two genetic conditions that are readily diagnosed through genetic testing. The specific mutations in DNA that cause the conditions are known, and it is possible to diagnose both disorders before a child is born and to counsel couples who carry the genetic mutations for future pregnancies. A proportion of children with both fragile X syn-drome and tuberous sclerosis develop autistic symptoms,[1] suggest-ing that the genes involved in causing these disorders may also be involved in causing ASD. Because it is now possible to identify single genes that are known to contribute to ASD in some cases, the American Academy of Pediatrics recommends that genetic testing be conducted on all individuals with a diagnosis of ASD. Two types of tests are done. One test, called *microarray analysis*, examines all of the individual chromosomes for mutated or miss-ing genes. The second test specifically tests for fragile X syndrome, one of the most common single-gene causes of ASD.

As mentioned earlier, there appear to be a variety of traits that run in the families of people with ASD, especially traits related to the areas of language and social abilities. Higher rates of language delay, articulation problems, learning difficulties, social difficul-ties, and social anxiety are found in relatives of people with ASD than in family members of people with other disabilities. Studies indicate that these milder difficulties show up in about 10–20% of siblings of individuals with ASD and often in parents as well.

---

[1] However, only a very small proportion of children with autism spectrum disorder have either fragile X syndrome or tuberous sclerosis. Some doctors routinely screen all children with ASD for these conditions, but others suggest genetic testing only if the child with ASD has certain physical features common in fragile X syndrome or tuberous sclerosis, as mentioned in Chapter 2.

The strengths of people with ASD can run in their families too. Parents and siblings often have talents and interests similar to those of people with ASDs. British researcher Simon Baron-Cohen proposed a theory that people in families with a member with an ASD would be especially skilled at understanding mechanical topics (such as how machines work), physical cause-and-effect mechanisms, and visual–spatial problems (as in puzzles). He and others have tested the theory that not only characteristic difficulties but also characteristic strengths run in families. Dr. Baron-Cohen's team found that the parents of children with ASD were more likely to be engineers, physicists, and mathematicians than the parents of other children (other scientists have also found elevated rates of accounting and science careers in families of individuals with ASD). Dr. Baron-Cohen's research group also surveyed over a thousand university students majoring either in literature or in math, physics, or engineering. They found that the rate of ASD was significantly higher in the families of the math, physics, or engineering students than in the families of the literature students. Finally, this British group of researchers tested the parents of children with ASD directly, giving them tests of both social understanding and visual–spatial skill. They found that the parents of students with ASDs were more skilled at solving puzzles and finding hidden shapes in complex drawings than control parents, as well as slightly less accurate than the other parents at interpreting the expressions on people's faces. Some more recent research projects have confirmed the finding that strong visual–spatial, mechanical, and memory skills are often found in the families of individuals with ASDs.

These findings all converge on one conclusion. What appears to be genetically transmitted in the families of people with ASD is not ASD per se, but a certain distinctive style of thinking about, relating to, and reacting to the world that brings with it both strengths and challenges. This underscores the future limits we envision in the ability to provide genetic counseling. If a person carries certain genes, it does not necessarily mean that he or she will have ASD. ASD may represent the most extreme outcome of the genes, but it may be just one of several possibilities, many of which are strengths. A further limitation in genetic counseling is that in some cases the genetic alteration that might have caused an individual to be vulnerable to ASD is not always inherited from the parent. Studies have found that sometimes these mutations occur spontaneously in the egg or sperm.

What about Environmental Causes?

Over the past several years, there has been increasing interest in understanding how the combination of genetic risk factors and environmental influences can increase risk for ASD. We will review some of these findings in this section. It is important to keep in mind that it is highly unlikely that one environmental risk factor, by itself, is the cause of an individual's ASD. Rather, several environmental factors, in combination with genetic risk factors, likely explain an individual's ASD. This has been likened to a bucket of water to which individual risk factors, represented as drops of water, are added. As these risk factors, or drops of water, accumulate, it finally reaches a threshold at which the water will overflow. Similarly, as the number of genetic and environmental risk factors increase for a given individual, the likelihood of reaching that threshold that results in ASD will increase. Thus, it is usually not possible to point to a single factor that explains why a given person develops ASD.

So what are some of the environmental factors that are associated with risk for ASD? Two factors have been associated with *decreased* risk for ASD. The first is being a female. Males are four to five times more likely to develop ASD than females. Studies suggest that being a female has a "protective" influence against genetic risk factors for ASD. It appears to take many more genetic "hits" before ASD develops if one is a female. The second factor associated with decreased risk for ASD is the mother's nutrition right before and during pregnancy. Specifically, taking prenatal vitamins, especially folic acid, has been associated with lower rates of ASD.

Although much of the research on environmental factors that might increase risk for ASD has only recently been published and needs to be replicated, a few findings are starting to emerge. One finding is that parents who are older when they conceive are slightly more likely to have a child with ASD. Although we don't know exactly why this is true, it is known that as we age, all of us accumulate tiny deletions in our chromosomes, and it is possible that this might contribute to increased risk for ASD. Recent studies suggest that exposure to high levels of toxins, such as air pollution, may be associated with increased risk for ASD. Also, certain pregnancy and birth complications are associated with increased risk for ASD. These include exposure to severe infections during pregnancy, such as the flu with high fever; being born prematurely with very low birthweight; and experiencing birth complications that restrict oxygen to the brain. It has also been suggested that such complications are not *causes* of autism but *consequences* of it. This interesting hypothesis speculates that obstetric problems may occur in pregnancies in which something has already gone wrong with fetal development. Evidence for this comes from children with genetic disorders like Down syndrome, whose mothers have higher than average rates of pregnancy and delivery complications. Down syndrome is determined at the moment of conception. Therefore, there is something different about the growing baby long before the obstetrical complications take place. Some scientists have wondered if a similar scenario could account for the slightly elevated rate of prenatal and birth difficulties seen in individuals with ASD. They reasoned that genetic factors, as discussed earlier in this chapter, act early in fetal development to in some way weaken or jeopardize the fetus so that the pregnancy and delivery fail to progress normally. In other words, the complications follow, rather than lead to, the ASD. As we mentioned earlier, none of these factors—by itself—is likely to explain a given child's ASD.

Rather, these factors have been shown to slightly increase the risk for ASD, especially in genetically vulnerable people.

In recent years, there has been increased interest in whether ASD could result from an inherited immune system deficiency that makes children more susceptible to viral or bacterial infections. Unable to clear the organism quickly, it has been hypothesized that the fetus or infant is at increased risk that the infection might damage the brain directly. Another possible mechanism is that early infections might trigger an *autoimmune response*, in which the body's immune system turns on itself and attacks its own parts as if they were foreign invaders (like viruses). It is thought that a similar breakdown of the immune system's "self-recognition" mechanisms leads to other autoimmune illnesses, such as diabetes. In diabetes, for example, the immune system is triggered by an infection, but instead of just fighting the virus or bacterium, it also attacks the body's own pancreas, killing the cells that produce insulin. The lack of insulin then causes the symptoms of diabetes. It has been proposed that some children with ASD might undergo such an autoimmune process, but that the organ of the body attacked by the immune system in the case of ASD is the brain rather than the pancreas. A few studies have found evidence of antibodies (immune proteins usually produced to combat infections) that "recognized" brain cells as "foreign" in some children with ASD. One further prediction of the autoimmunity theory is that children with ASD should have a higher rate of other autoimmune illnesses, such as asthma, allergies, arthritis, diabetes, multiple sclerosis, and the like. Some studies have indeed found an elevated rate of some of these difficulties in both children with ASD and their family members.

The environmental factors discussed above are ones that could potentially influence the development of the fetus during pregnancy. One factor that would have an influence later in a child's development that has received much interest and controversy is vaccines, especially the measles–mumps–rubella (MMR) vaccine that is administered at about the time that some children with ASD regress and develop symptoms. The many studies that have been conducted to date do not support this hypothesis.

This chapter has discussed a wide range of potential causes for ASD, including genetic and environmental risk factors. There are many different ways for an individual to end up with ASD. Even when causes are found, each cause will apply only to a small group of children. New theories are generated every few months, some of which prove to be fruitful and others of which lead to dead ends. Parents often ask if they should have new medical tests performed as new theories about cause appear. Typically, doctors suggest waiting, because it will take time for a useful theory explaining ASD to evolve, as research centers around the world tackle the question. The search for answers is a universal human need that affects both parents and scientists, so there is no doubt that the search for causes will continue and intensify in the future.

4

Treatments for High-Functioning Autism Spectrum Disorder

As Seth's parents heard the psychologist say "autism spectrum disorder," they were worried about what the future would hold for them and their son. "Fortunately," the psychologist continued, "there are some very good programs that have been developed to treat the exact kinds of challenges Seth has." She handed them a slip of paper with a phone number written on it and encouraged them to call that very afternoon, saying, "They will give you the tools you need to help Seth." Seth enrolled in a preschool that was designed to help children with ASD that fall. He stayed in this program for 2 years, until he was eligible for kindergarten. His parents asked his teachers what type of program he should be enrolled in next, and were delighted but a little worried by their reply: "Children like Seth can usually function quite well in a regular classroom after this." While Seth had made rapid progress in preschool and could now talk very well, he still had many difficulties, and his parents knew that his need for special services was far from over. Thus began their long search for therapies, programs, and classes that would help their bright, talkative, but socially challenged son negotiate his course through life.

So Now What?

Obtaining a diagnosis may not be the most important outcome of your child's assessment. Even more critical is what the diagnosis tells you about how to help your child develop the skills needed to be successful in school, with peers, and beyond. The rest of this book covers methods of addressing specific challenges associated with ASD while capitalizing on the strengths associated with high-functioning ASD. This chapter presents an overview of the different treatment options available in many communities and, when known, their relative benefits and risks. As discussed in Chapter 1, the range of outcomes seen in adolescents and adults with ASD is wide. All children make progress with treatment. Some people quickly improve a great deal and their disabilities become less apparent over time. They function well in a variety of different roles and settings typical for their age—college student, employee, roommate, friend, neighbor—with few apparent impairments. Others continue to face significant challenges, but nevertheless are able to live productive and happy lives with some support. In this chapter you'll learn which currently available treatments seem to maximize the likelihood of the best outcome for your individual child. We hope that as more children are diagnosed and treated early, it will be easier for them to succeed well in adolescence and adulthood.

While treatments for ASD are becoming more available in many communities, you may have to do a good deal of the tracking down and setting up of your child's therapies yourself. As you'll realize while reading this chapter, there is a fairly long list of interventions that may help your child. *Some* of these approaches will benefit *some* children, but very *few* (if any) will help *all* children. Even tried-and-true treatments for common medical illnesses, like aspirin and antibiotics, are not effective for everyone and may even be harmful for some people. ASD and its treatments are no different. Only very rarely are the different treatments described in this chapter offered under one roof, by one agency, clinic, or therapist.

This is the bad news that comes with the good news that your child is more mildly affected by ASD. Unlike programs for children with moderate-to-severe ASD, there are fewer comprehensive programs that address all the needs of the higher-functioning child. You will need to find a professional who can help you assess your child's specific skills and deficits and draw up an individualized treatment plan. There is limited research to indicate which children are most likely to benefit from which therapy—choosing a therapy is based on the clinical recommendations of your evaluator, availability, and your preferences. And then it is necessary to monitor progress and determine whether the therapy is working or whether other options should be explored. You will become an expert in your child's abilities and disabilities, making decisions about which of the treatments to try and educating teachers, service providers, and others about your child. You will become your child's best advocate. In some ways, this is a less-than-ideal situation, because you are likely already experiencing a tremendous amount of stress while parenting your special child and supporting and raising a family. But there are no teachers, therapists, or agencies that can be available to your child 24 hours a day, 7 days a week, for the rest of his or her life. You are the consistent thread from one classroom to another, from one intervention to another, from one therapist to another, who manages all the details, remembers all the important facts, and knows what worked and what didn't. You will be heavily involved in teaching your child how to learn new skills and respond in everyday situations when therapists or teachers are not present. You are a critical ingredient in your child's life. The rest of this chapter, and this book, will give you the resources, skills, and support to succeed in this role while minimizing the tremendous burden it can represent.

"When Julie was diagnosed with ASD when she was 3, we knew very little about ASD and were unsure where to turn and what to do. Julie was so smart, even precocious, so at first we wondered if the diagnosis was wrong. But her constant repetition of dialogue from Disney videos and difficulties interacting with others fit autism to a tee. So we both took a deep breath and vowed we'd do everything we could to help Julie. It was confusing and daunting at first. The Internet was full of information about 'miraculous' and sometimes expensive treatments. It was paralyzing at first. How could we know which treatment would work best for Julie? Which treatments were worth investing our time and money in? Eventually, we found trusted people—both other parents and professionals—who helped guide us through these early months. We've decided to concentrate on what we can do to help our daughter make the best of who she is. And the future looks brighter than we could have guessed a year ago. ASD will likely always be a part of Julie's life. And that's not necessarily a bad thing. ASD is part of what makes Julie the unique and special person she is."

Treatment Options in the Preschool Years

If you have a preschool child who was recently diagnosed with ASD, you have several treatment options. Some of these have received much media attention, and you may already be aware of them. What you probably don't know is whether they are as appropriate for your high-functioning child. Research suggests that all children on the autism spectrum, regardless of functional level, benefit from intensive early intervention. In fact, children with ASD who have stronger cognitive and language skills are the most likely to make rapid progress in response to early intervention. Research has now shown that early intervention can actually stimulate brain regions that are responsible for social behavior, leading to rewiring, reorganization, and the formation of new neural connections important for appropriate social behavior and communication. Additionally, your child's strong cognitive and language skills will help your child develop strategies that can compensate for skills that your child may find difficult to acquire. For example, he can use his strong memory skills to memorize rules and scripts that are useful for social interaction.

Some parents and professionals wonder whether children who are bright, verbal, and relatively more interested in social interaction should receive intensive early intervention. In most cases, such interventions are the best choice for achieving optimal outcomes. Depending on the services available in your own community, this may mean that you will decide to enroll your child in a home- or center-based preschool program specifically designed for children with special needs such as ASD. This investment in intensive early intervention will pay off later and provide the best chance for your child to function in less restrictive or specialized educational classrooms when older.

It is important to understand that your child has the right to inclusion in the least restrictive educational setting in which your child is able to make progress. You, as parents, will have your own opinions about what classroom is best, which may differ from those of the doctors working with your child. What you should know as you choose treatment programs for your child is that multiple intermediate options exist, in addition to the two extremes of a specialized self-contained program versus a regular classroom. For example, some parents enroll their child in a self-contained special education program, but then also have the child attend the neighborhood school for a regular preschool class or for social or extracurricular activities, perhaps with the assistance of an aide. Another option is to administer the early intervention treatments in a regular preschool classroom, rather than at home or in a special education setting. This is a good option if the regular education teacher is flexible and will allow other specialists to participate in the classroom or even use some of the intervention strategies herself. Many parents will feel comfortable starting off with a more intensive early intervention program, delivered at home or in a special classroom setting, when their child is young, to ensure that the child gains the skills necessary to be educated in a regular education classroom by the time kindergarten starts. More important than the setting is that your child receive high-quality intervention that is sensitive to your child's unique learning style, strengths, and challenges, and that your child is making good progress and thriving well in the setting you have chosen.

Depending on where you live, some of the following interventions may be more popular or more available than others. Currently, these approaches are the most widely accepted and most effective preschool interventions. More information on each of them, as well as other treatment options, can be found in the Resources at the back of the book. Table 3 also compares their features.

Autism Speaks (*www.autismspeaks.org*) provides a comprehensive list of various early intervention approaches, along with videotapes that demonstrate each one. This will help you decide which approach might be the best fit for your child. Although some of these treatments have more scientific evidence to back them up than others, there have been very few studies that have compared two different treatments to see which is the more effective. Furthermore, all studies that have evaluated the effectiveness of the available early intervention models have found that some children respond dramatically and quickly and others make slower progress. In other words, there is no "one-approach-fits-all" solution. Depending on your child's unique strengths, unique challenges, and unique learning style, as well as the availability of treatments (and associated costs) in your community, you will need to decide for yourself what works best. Then, by monitoring whether your child is making progress and thriving in the classroom or treatment model you chose, you will be able to determine whether changes or tweaks to the program are needed. These changes and tweaks are inevitable because the needs of your child will change over time.

Although research has not clarified the optimal number of hours of treatment a child should receive, generally at least 25 hours of structured intervention each week are recommended dur-

TABLE 3. Treatments for ASD

Treatment	Ages	How and where delivered	Features	Strengths and weaknesses
Applied behavior analysis (ABA)	Preschool	Usually but not always at home, by a trained professional team, 20–40 hours a week	One-on-one teaching of basic social, communication, attention, and academic skills, using behavioral principles of positive consequences (rewards) for desirable behavior and negative consequences for undesirable behavior	Costly if insurance doesn't cover, but allows many children with 2 years of treatment to function well in regular school without special support
Early Start Denver Model (ESDM)	Infancy (12 months) through late preschool age	At home and school	Uses ABA strategies and also emphasizes play, positive social relationships, child-preferred activities, sharing emotions with others	Studies demonstrate effectiveness in increasing language, IQ, and social skills
Treatment and Education of Autistic and related Communication-handicapped CHildren (TEACCH)	Preschool to adulthood	Mainly at school, with home supplementation possible, by teachers and parents	Visual structure and organization of environment and learning materials using visual, mechanical, and memory strengths to teach language, imitation, social, and cognitive skills; one-on-one or in groups	Outcome less well studied than ABA and ESDM
Social skills groups	Preschool through adulthood	Therapist's office, clinic, or school, led by therapist or teacher	Development of conversational skills, body language, perspective taking, reading of others' emotions, regulating emotions, social problem-solving skills such as dealing with being teased or left out	Teaches skills and provides practice with peers; provides tools that translate to home training; can be used through adulthood

(continued)

Treatment	Ages	How and where delivered	Features	Strengths and weaknesses
Educational support	Preschool through college	School	Accommodations to and modifications of environment and academic goals	Negotiable with schools; adaptable to individual needs; mandated by federal laws
Pragmatic language–communication therapy	Preschool through adulthood	Group setting or pairs of children, provided by speech–language pathologist	Training in pragmatics of language: social communication, abstract or complex language concepts	Beneficial when social skills group is unavailable or when child has more communication problems
Functional behavior analysis	Preschool through adulthood	School, home, and other settings, by any adult in charge	Examination of function of disruptive or problem behaviors; provision of more appropriate ways to communicate	Reduces behavior problems and increases communication skills
Medication	All ages	Prescribed by a medical doctor, such as a pediatrician, child psychiatrist, or neurologist; given usually daily by parents at home	Alters levels of brain chemicals that are affecting child's behavior	May be helpful for attention or activity level problems, depression, anxiety, anger, but does not treat social or communication symptoms of ASD
Sensory integration therapy	Preschool, childhood	Office of an occupational therapist, possibly with home exercises provided	Decreases sensory sensitivities, develops coping skills and tolerance for new sensations	Little research to determine effectiveness
Individual psychotherapy	Adolescence through adulthood	Office of a psychotherapist, potentially with "trips" into community	Explores moods and emotional states; develops self-awareness and self-acceptance; takes a cognitive-behavioral approach	Best for individuals with good insight; may not generalize to group settings; needs to be as directive and concrete as possible

ing the preschool years. This can include a range of treatments, such as participation in a regular or special preschool program, speech–language therapy, and occupational therapy, in addition to early behavioral intervention. Parents' use of intervention strategies at home counts as well. The point here is that typically developing children have many opportunities for learning throughout the day, and we want to ensure that children with ASD are also having many learning opportunities. How many hours and types of services should be delivered often is based on the child's readiness, rate of progress, and response to treatment and the child's need for rest and other family activities, as well as community standards and the range of local services available. Because of the intensity of the program, school systems may not have an autism-specific early intervention program in place. If you and your doctors believe early intensive behavioral intervention is the appropriate intervention, you may have to work with your local school district to develop the program for your child. Here are descriptions of a few of the most commonly used early intervention approaches:

Applied Behavior Analysis

In the 1960s, Dr. Ivar Lovaas as well as other psychologists began using a method called applied behavior analysis (ABA). Lovaas then went on to develop a model of early intervention that used a teaching method called discrete trial training, sometimes called the "Lovaas method." The Lovaas/ABA method uses general principles of behavioral therapy to build the skills that children with ASD lack, such as language, play, self-help, social, academic, and attentional skills. In addition, this model incorporates strategies to minimize the unusual and repetitive behaviors of autism spectrum disorder.

In the Lovaas model, teaching is initially done one-on-one and is highly individualized, with specific treatment goals chosen based on the child's abilities and challenges. Once basic communication, social, and attention skills are mastered, the child is gradually introduced into a group learning situation. A member of the treatment team at first accompanies the child to the classroom to facilitate transfer of skills between the two settings. The aide, or "shadow," is eventually faded from the class, and the child is then fully integrated into the regular school program. This process may take 2 or more years to complete, and many children are able to attend a general classroom by kindergarten.

Spencer's parents heard about a promising educational program based on ABA principles from an acquaintance whose son also had ASD. They were referred to a local psychologist trained in the use of ABA, who did some testing with Spencer to determine his individual needs. After concluding that Spencer would likely benefit from early intensive behavioral intervention, the psychologist recommended that a home program consisting of approximately a dozen goals be set up. Since Spencer was bright and already had some useful skills (talking in simple sentences, sitting in a chair, and attending), the initial goals were primarily academic: identifying colors, shapes, numbers, and letters; stating the functions of objects; answering questions ("What is your name?"; "How old are you?"); identifying environmental sounds; imitating two-step sequences; and drawing shapes. Communication and social goals were also incorporated, such as how to have a brief conversation and greet others. Therapists came into his home daily to work with him, and Spencer progressed rapidly. Within only a few months, he had mastered all of his initial goals. Spencer's parents also noticed changes in his behavior: his eye contact was better, he talked in longer sentences, and he was more cooperative at home and in his church nursery school. As Spencer progressed, new goals were added to increase his pretend play skills, his ability to ask questions and make comments, and his ability to take turns and follow rules of simple games. Over the following year, Spencer continued to improve, so his intervention team decided that he was ready for some integration into a regular preschool to work on his skills with peers. He began attending 4 hours a week, with an aide helping him. Time in the preschool was gradually increased to 15 hours. By the time he was 5, his parents felt ready to enroll Spencer in a regular kindergarten class without any special assistance. He still had a few quirks, but he seemed as bright and ready for kindergarten as any other child in their neighborhood. They finally breathed a sigh of relief when Spencer's kindergarten teacher told them what a delightful son they had. She commented that he was academically advanced and chuckled about his habit of asking all the adults what their license plate number was.

Research has demonstrated that many children, especially those who are high functioning, who begin treatment early and receive 2 years of ABA-based treatment are able to enter and function well in typical first-grade classrooms, without special support. In addition, Lovaas's study found that the cognitive abilities of treated children (as measured by standardized tests) were far higher than those of untreated children with ASD. So it's no surprise that ABA-based interventions are very popular in many areas. An obvious drawback, however, is the expense and effort of one-on-one treatment. Almost none of the children that Lovaas's team studied who had received only 10 hours a week or less of ABA model treatment achieved the same success as the kids who had 40 hours a week of treatment. Information about early intervention providers using ABA methods in your region is available from the Autism Speaks website (*www.autismspeaks.org/resource-guide/by-state*). The national organization called FEAT (Families for Early Autism Treatment) also maintains a web page that lists ABA providers by state (*www.feat.org*).

Early Start Denver Model

Another option for early intervention is the Early Start Denver Model (ESDM) developed by Drs. Sally Rogers and Geraldine Dawson. ESDM can be used with children as young as 12 months of age. This approach incorporates the principles of ABA but also emphasizes the parent–child relationship as a foundation for learning. Teaching occurs in the context of play-based activities in which language, communication, social behaviors, and cognitive skills are taught. Like traditional ABA, ESDM has been validated in research studies and shown to lead to increases in cognitive, language, and social skills. ESDM can also be delivered by parents at home. In a study published in 2010, it was found that children who received the ESDM intervention for 15 hours per week for 2 years made significant gains in IQ, language, adaptive behavior, and social skills. The manual is available in many languages, including Spanish.

Strategies based on the ESDM model that parents can use to promote language, social interaction, and learning are described in the book *An Early Start for Your Child with Autism*, by Sally Rogers, Geraldine Dawson, and Laurie Vismara. You can use these strategies in combination with treatment provided by a therapist or even begin them while you are waiting to be enrolled in an intervention program. These are strategies that promote communication, social engagement, and learning that can be used during your regularly daily activities with your child, such as during meals, bathtime, and play activities.

TEACCH

Another treatment approach in use in some parts of the United States and around the world is the TEACCH model (this acronym stands for the Treatment and Education of Autistic and related Communication-handicapped CHildren program). This treatment program was developed in the 1960s by Dr. Eric Schopler, a psychologist at the University of North Carolina. A cornerstone of the TEACCH educational approach is visual structure and organization of the environment and learning materials. As discussed in Chapter 2, many children with ASD have difficulty with abstract, language-based tasks and instructional techniques but have relatively strong visual–spatial capacities. The TEACCH program capitalizes on the visual, mechanical, and rote memory strengths of many children with ASD, using them to develop more challenging skills, such as language, imitation, cognitive, and social skills.

TEACCH programs typically structure academic, social, communication, and imitation tasks for the child so that what is expected and how to complete it are visually apparent. Visual schedules, consisting of pictures and words that show daily events in order of occurrence, help the child anticipate what is to come or the work that needs to be done during a teaching session. The child can then, on her own, without teacher prompts, "predict the future." Many children with ASD tend to tantrum or become upset when things in their environment change. They cling to the familiar, not necessarily because they enjoy what they are doing but because they *know* what they are doing and *don't know* what comes next. Introduction of a picture schedule can significantly reduce anxiety, frustration, and tantrums, in addition to promoting more independent functioning. See the Resources for information on how to order materials to be used in making visual schedules. While outcomes of children participating in TEACCH interventions have not been examined as closely as outcomes for other treatments discussed so far in the chapter, parents and professionals often choose to combine elements of the TEACCH model (such as visual schedules) with elements of other intervention programs, integrating treatments to best meet the needs of an individual child.

Seth's preschool teachers implemented a schedule for him after seeing how anxious and upset he became when there were changes to his school day and how much he thrived on routines. When Seth memorized what was coming up (for example, lunch immediately follows a trip to the bathroom and washing hands), he was eager to move on to the next activity. However, even minor deviations in the routine, such as staying indoors on a rainy day, elicited shrieks of dismay from Seth, followed by many minutes of lying on the floor, kicking at anyone who approached. His teachers decided to begin using a schedule for Seth, which showed in pictures each of the major events of his day (see Figure 2). When something wasn't going to take place as usual, they used the universal "no" sign (red circle with a slash through it) to indicate the change. They were amazed when Seth's tantrums quickly stopped. He was even able to take it in stride when his speech therapy was canceled due to his therapist's illness, as long as his teacher indicated the change on the schedule.

These are a few of the most commonly used approaches to early intervention. Additional approaches are described on the Autism Speaks website (*www.autismspeaks.org*). The doctor who diagnosed your child will probably also have a list of community treatment referrals available, as may your community mental health center or the psychiatry departments of local hospitals. Federal law requires that every child who has delays in development be offered services, which are referred to as "Part C—Birth to Three Services" for children below 3 years of age and "Part B—Preschool Services." Your pediatrician should provide you with a contact number so you can find and obtain these services, at no cost.

As you consider which option is best for your child, keep in mind that, at present, however, no studies have directly compared the different treatment approaches just described. Thus, which programs have the most benefit for which children is not certain.

Seth's Schedule

FIGURE 2. Visual schedules can be used to decrease anxiety and promote independent functioning. The picture communication symbols used in Seth's schedule are ©1981/2014 by DynaVox Mayer-Johnson LLC. All Rights Reserved Worldwide. Used with permission.

We recommend that you find the options available in your community, visit and observe the therapists or schools offering them, discuss them with your doctor, and weigh the costs and benefits to both your child and your family before making treatment decisions.

Interventions for Preschool and Beyond

If the preschool program your child attends is intensive and comprehensive, then you may not have the time or the need for the following treatments until he is older. But what if you missed the preschool years and the interventions just discussed? What if your child was diagnosed after age 5? Or what if, like Seth's parents, you've found a very effective preschool program and want to continue with some interventions upon entering grade school? All is not lost! A wide variety of helpful interventions are available for older children. As mentioned earlier, they may not always be easy to find or readily offered to your child, but they *are* out there.

Some of these interventions use the same principles as the preschool programs just reviewed, so your child may still benefit from the use of behavioral or visual techniques, at a level appropriate for her age and developmental level. The two most common needs of children with higher-functioning ASD are social skills training and educational assistance. There is a wide variety of different interventions for each, so we have devoted a separate chapter to each of these topics and will mention them only briefly here.

Treatment needs vary widely from child to child, but we have listed the following interventions roughly in order from the most to the least commonly needed.

Social Interventions

By now you certainly know that difficulties in the social realm are among the most prominent of the problems faced by your child. Naturally, therefore, they are an important domain for intervention. The many options for working on social behavior are discussed in more detail in Chapter 8. Social skills groups are one option that can be a particularly helpful resource. These groups focus explicitly on the social behaviors that other children seem to learn naturally. We can't take for granted that children with ASD will absorb and imitate typical social behaviors just by being around others who perform them naturally (siblings, parents, peers). Social behavior is best taught in a social setting, and social skills groups provide that setting, along with the structure needed to teach these complex skills. Some common topics that such groups address include appropriate body language and eye contact, reading the emotions of others, and taking others' perspectives. Conversational skills and other behaviors important to interactions, such as introducing oneself, joining a group, giving compliments, negotiating, sharing, and taking turns, are a typical focus of social skills groups. Additionally, they usually address social problem-solving skills, such as handling teasing and being told "no," dealing with being left out, and regulating and expressing emotions in age-appropriate ways. A benefit of this approach is that your child has the chance to try out these skills in a safe situation, hopefully providing the opportunity to have social "fun" and increase the child's motivation to improve these skills. Research has shown that social skills interventions are effective for improving children's abilities to play, make friends, handle teasing, and manage a wide range of social situations. Often these interventions take place in a group setting and are offered at school and at local clinics. Speech–language therapists sometimes offer social skills training.

A related type of intervention relies on video modeling. Research has shown that this approach is effective for teaching social skills to children with ASD. The approaches use video recording to display a model of the targeted behavior or social skill. Typically, it involves recording a person modeling the target skills. The child views the video and then practices the targeted behavior. This approach takes advantage of the strong visual skills of many children with ASD. Video modeling can be used while working one-on-one with a child or in a group setting as part of social skills training.

Your area may not have a social skills group exclusively for children with ASD, but there may well be one for children with attentional or other behavior problems. The child or adolescent with ASD often benefits from the opportunity to meet other kids with ASD who share similar interests, personality styles, temperaments, and challenges. But as long as the group addresses many of the issues listed above and you feel that there is a good fit between the therapeutic goals of the group and your child's needs, it is not necessary that all or even most of the participants have ASD. You should also check with your school district, since social skills groups may be offered through schools.

There are also several things you can do around your home or community to improve your child's social behavior and provide opportunities to practice social skills:

- Write out "scripts" that help your child know what to do and say in certain social situations, such as answering the telephone or ordering food in a restaurant.
- Videotape your child having a conversation with someone and then watch it together, pointing out both things he or she did well and things that need improvement.
- Videotape others (perhaps siblings) to provide a model of age-appropriate conversation.
- Enroll your child in groups that revolve around his or her special interests so that he or she has an opportunity to meet like-minded others.
- Invite peers to the home to play and then carefully monitor the interactions and provide structure and support to help your child learn turn taking, sharing, compromising, and other skills.
- Set aside 15 minutes each day in which you converse with your child, uninterrupted by siblings, household chores, or

the telephone, about a prearranged set of topics (school, plans for the weekend, jokes). You might furnish the topics to your child beforehand or have them written down to encourage sticking to the topics and discourage drifting to your child's special interests. If needed, you might provide visual cues that encourage turn taking (perhaps an arrow that can be pointed toward the person whose turn it is to speak) and discourage verbosity (for example, a stop sign that can be held up to indicate that your child is going on too long).

These and many other techniques used in both clinic and home settings to improve social behavior are described in more detail in Chapter 8.

Educational Assistance

The second area of typical need is educational support. Despite average or better intelligence, many students with ASD have difficulty in school or don't achieve at the level expected. They have difficulty organizing and regulating themselves in class and managing time, often resulting in failure to complete work during school and many extra hours of homework. They may have trouble planning ahead, setting appropriate goals and subgoals, estimating the time it takes to complete tasks, and remembering to bring home what is needed to complete homework assignments. These problems with self-regulation, goal selection, and attention may result in spells of daydreaming or absorption in inner thoughts. Inflexibility and rigid problem-solving strategies also affect school performance. Finally, children with ASD are often not motivated by the same kinds of rewards that other children are. They do not particularly care that their teachers or parents will be displeased if they leave work unfinished or get poor grades. They may have little intrinsic motivation to work on topics that aren't related to things that interest them. They may care little if they get detentions or have to stay in from recess; for a child stressed by social interactions, these punishments might actually be rewarding! Therefore, it can be difficult to inspire the child with ASD to do schoolwork, even when her intellectual abilities are strong.

For these reasons, most children with ASD will need some classroom accommodations and modifications to succeed in school. There may also need to be some adjustment of academic goals, perhaps placing more or less emphasis on certain subjects, making work more or less challenging than that of classmates, or making schoolwork more directly functional. For example, you may want more emphasis placed on vocational and daily living skills than on a traditional academic curriculum. It may be necessary to start working on these skills earlier than would be typical for other children to promote your child's ability to live independently and function in a work setting as an adult. Year-round schools or academic summer programs are often helpful, because change is difficult for most children with ASD and they can regress in behavior and academic skills over the long summer vacation.

In Chapter 7, we describe in detail the kinds of educational supports and services that appear most useful for students with ASD. Many of the accommodations we suggest capitalize on your child's good visual skills and memory, using these strengths to make up for weaknesses in organization, planning, attention, and flexibility. The most essential part of educational programming is adapting the curriculum to your child's individual problems and unique abilities (more on this topic in Chapter 5 as well). At this point we will say only that, in addition to finding social skills training for your child, you will probably want to contact your school district to discuss the most appropriate ways to deliver educational support to your child.

Pragmatic Language–Communication Therapy

Most individuals with milder ASD have relatively well-developed language abilities. They can speak fluently, in full sentences, with few or no grammatical errors. Yet they most likely exhibit some difficulty using language in a social context to exchange ideas and information with others. They usually have trouble with abstract or complex language concepts. When what we say isn't exactly what we mean (such as when we are sarcastic, joking, or using metaphors or other figures of speech), the child with ASD may misunderstand. All these difficulties are collectively referred to as deficits in the "pragmatics" of language. There are rules that underlie conversation that the rest of us learn naturally and know implicitly. These include taking turns, providing enough information to be clear without being verbose, and contributing relevant information. We know how to choose appropriate topics, how to stay on a topic, and how to switch to a new subject. We know how to "read" other people and can adjust our communication to the needs of the person with whom we are speaking. If someone seems bored, we try to liven up our conversation or change topics. If someone seems confused, we try to figure out why and provide clarification. We speak differently to a child than to an authority figure or a peer. We understand how intonation or an accompanying facial expression can change the meaning of what we say. However, children with ASD may not know these rules and often have to be taught them explicitly.

Much of this can be addressed in a good social skills group. (After all, how do we separate communication from social skills? The two go hand-in-hand.) But if no such group is available in your area or if the group does not address such conversational skills, you may want to explore whether some form of speech–language therapy would be helpful for your child. Ask around to find a speech–language pathologist experienced in working with people with ASD. Find out whether the person offers "pragmatic language" training or therapy in conversational skills. Often such therapy is offered in a group setting or with at least two children present. These skills are not well remediated in isolation, with just a therapist and your child present. Most children with ASD perform well in such structured situations, where the demands are lower and the conversational partner is forgiving. These skills need to be practiced with other children, with the guidance of a knowledgeable therapist who can provide a supportive atmosphere and explicit feedback about the strengths and weaknesses of the child's communication style.

Behavioral Interventions to Address Challenging Behaviors

Children and adolescents with ASD can demonstrate some unusual and problematic behaviors that require specific management. Your child may at times have temper outbursts, meltdowns, or tantrums that seem out of proportion to the incident (or are unpredictable, with no apparent trigger). Or maybe your child is impulsive and distractible, shouting out in class, grabbing things from other people, or having trouble sitting and focusing on work. Perhaps your child is very rigid about routines, the order in which things are done, or where favorite objects are placed. One young boy named Mark insisted that boxes of cereal be eaten in order by weight—that is, if the Cheerios box weighed more than the Rice Krispies box, it had to be completely consumed before the next box of cereal could be opened. Josh, a 15-year-old with ASD, knows a lot about presidents and likes to be "quizzed" about presidential facts—if, however, he gets an answer wrong, he insists that the person quizzing him start over with the first question and repeat every single one in order, until he gets to the question he got wrong. This is accompanied by a lot of shouting and crying, as Josh becomes very distressed when he is corrected. All of these issues can be dealt with by using *behavioral methods*, treatments that rely on principles of applied behavior analysis to teach more appropriate behavior. Behavioral strategies can be classified in two broad categories, those that modify behavior by changing what *precedes* the behavior and those that modify behavior by changing the *consequences* of the behavior.

Changing What Precedes the Behavior

The first approach can be thought of as a preventive approach. It is meant to stop behavior problems before they start, by changing things in the environment that are known to cause disruption, anxiety, or other stress to the child with ASD. Many of the strategies described in Chapter 7 regarding classroom accommodations fall into this category. We encourage educators to teach the child using visual methods and to provide as much structure and organization as possible. This capitalization on the strengths and minimization of the weaknesses known to be associated with ASD is just one example of the preventive approach to behavior management. Other examples include being sure that your child is well rested and not hungry, making sure that the side effects of medications are not causing behavior problems, and using visual schedules to increase predictability and consistency for your child. All these "interventions" are intended to decrease stress on your child and increase his feelings of control, and thus may be effective in reducing behavior problems.

Changing the Consequences of Behavior

The second strategy, providing specific consequences to mold appropriate behavior, derives from operant conditioning theory, made famous by Dr. B. F. Skinner. Most living things, from the simplest invertebrates to humans, from infants to adults, and from those with ASD to those without, can change their behavior based on these learning principles. Specifically, if a behavior is *reinforced*, that is, followed by something good, then it increases in frequency, while if it is punished, ignored, or followed by any other negative outcome, it decreases in frequency. We can use these principles to change the behavior of children with ASD (in fact, ABA therapy, described above, is based on these very principles). If there are things we want to teach, we reinforce them. If there are behaviors we want to go away, we provide negative consequences for them. Most people with ASD learn well when provided with explicit rules. Reward systems can be set up that make it worth the child's while to follow the rules. Obviously, rewards that are effective incentives for children with ASD are likely to be those linked with the child's particular area of intense interest, such as extra time looking up dragonflies on the Internet, a trip to the zoo exclusively to see the insect displays, and the like. But your child may appreciate other, more generic rewards, just like other kids, whether they are favorite dinners or special privileges such as staying up later than usual. Experiment, just like you would with your "typical" children. But before you come up with either rewards or punishments, be sure to explore preventive strategies, because some problem behaviors can be eliminated altogether through changes in the environment and other forms of structure. If this does not eliminate the problem or result in the desired behavior, an operant approach may be successful.

Jenna is a young girl with ASD who had resisted sleeping alone since infancy. She would cry and tantrum when put down in her own bed, but would easily fall asleep in her parents' bed. They would then carry her back to her own bed. However, later in the night she would awaken, wander through the house, line up favorite items, help herself to food from the refrigerator, and eventually climb back into her parents' bed to sleep for the rest of the night. When her parents woke one night to find Jenna sitting up in between them with a library book and a pair of scissors, they decided to seek help. They first went to their doctor to explore whether there might be some physical reason, like seizures, that could be contributing to Jenna's night waking. After ruling this out, as well as making some changes in her diet (eliminating food and drinks with any caffeine and decreasing liquid intake in the evenings) that did not change her sleep, they were referred to a psychologist.

A behavioral program was set up that included clear rules for Jenna to follow and clear rewards for doing so. A bedtime routine was established that consisted of putting on pajamas, brushing teeth, using the toilet, reading two books, saying prayers, turning out the light, kisses and hugs, closing the door halfway, and then parents leaving the room. A photo of Jenna engaging in each of these steps was taken and placed in order on a piece of cardboard that was then taped next to her bed. The sentence JENNA, STAY IN YOUR BED was written on the bottom of the chart. Jenna, with her parents' help, made a list of all the things she would like to earn for staying in bed, including favorite snacks (which were withheld at other times of the day), small trinkets and toys, special activities with Mom and Dad (making cookies, going on a walk around the neighborhood, playing a game), access to favorite videos, and so forth. Each was written on a piece of paper and then put in a box covered with question marks.

Jenna was given a progressive schedule for earning these rewards, which she accessed by pulling a slip of paper from the "mystery" box. For the first week, she could earn a reward just by cooperatively following the beginning parts of the bedtime routine schedule. In the second week, she could earn a reward by staying in bed without crying for 1 minute; she was then permitted to sleep in her parents' bed as usual. This time was gradually lengthened, and Jenna could earn the reward only by staying in bed for longer and longer periods of time. Eventually she began to fall asleep while lying in her bed; then the required behavior for the reward became staying in bed throughout the night.

While it took many weeks for Jenna to reach the eventual goal, this procedure was successful in gradually shaping her sleep patterns so that they conformed with the behavior desired by her parents. Jenna greatly looked forward to her rewards and seemed to be highly motivated by the mystery involved in not knowing exactly what she would earn. Jenna's parents gradually lengthened the interval between the behavior and the rewards (for example, she needed to sleep in her own bed each night for a week to earn one) until Jenna seemed to have forgotten all about the rewards and had firmly established the new behavior.

The plan to help Jenna sleep in her own bed has several important ingredients to highlight. Her parents first explored *possible causes* of the problem, such as seizures and caffeine intake, and made environmental changes. Then they established a behavioral plan that had *clear, predictable rules* that were provided to Jenna in a *visual format*. They made sure that the *rewards were actually reinforcing* to Jenna by having her choose them. The requirements for reinforcement were at first set very low, so that Jenna experienced *immediate success*. There was a *gradual shaping of behavior* and a *gradual fading of rewards*, so that Jenna had to work harder over time to earn reinforcement, and expectations were slowly made more age-appropriate.

If necessary, negative consequences can be added to such a behavioral plan. Jenna's parents did not find it necessary to do this, but they could have added another component to the plan indicating what would happen if Jenna did not achieve the specified goal. For example, in addition to not earning the desired reward, she might have lost some small privilege if she got out of bed (5 minutes' less television the next evening). We talk more about methods for dealing with challenging behavior in Chapter 6.

Methods like this can also be used to reduce obsessive or repetitive behavior. The key ingredients to all such plans include exploring contributing factors in the environment, setting up explicit rules and consequences, consistently adhering to them, and increasing demands in a stepwise fashion so that change is introduced gradually. Dr. Patricia Howlin, a British psychologist who has worked with people with ASD for many years, described using these principles to gradually decrease a young boy's obsession with "Thomas the Tank Engine" trains. A picture calendar was made that showed when access to the trains was allowed. Less popular "Thomas" activities were substituted for more preferred ones (such as reading a "Thomas" book rather than watching a video). Engaging in alternate activities was strongly rewarded as reinforcement for "Thomas"-related activities was withdrawn.

Sometimes it is not enough to simply provide consequences for behavior and expect it to change. If the behavior serves a very important purpose, then it may persist no matter how many rewards or punishments are introduced. Let's say, for example, that a child continually interrupts and yells out comments and repetitive questions during class. If the child needs more attention from her teacher and is obtaining it by yelling and interrupting, then the behavior will be very hard to change until an equally powerful alternative is given to the child to obtain the desired attention. If the child is given a hand gesture or written sign that she can use instead, and the teacher learns to consistently respond to the signal, then the interrupting behavior may go away without any need for a behavioral system of rewards. Likewise, if a child gets agitated and begins hitting himself during class, an examination of the function of the behavior may indicate that the child is trying to communicate that a task is too difficult. If an alternative way of expressing this frustration and desire to change activities is found (for example, giving the teacher a card with a picture of a stop sign on it), the self-hitting may stop abruptly. Problem behaviors can serve many functions; in addition to getting attention or escaping from an unpleasant task, they might indicate a need for help, a need to obtain a desired object, or boredom. Chapter 6 contains advice on puzzling through the possible messages your child is trying to convey with problematic behavior. Finding alternate ways to communicate these messages and ultimately to solve the problems behind them is at the heart of this type of behavioral intervention, called *functional behavior analysis*, also discussed further in Chapter 6. Psychologists and educators use a variety of assessment tools to discover the functions of behavior and then change them. If your child is having such problems, ask a behaviorally oriented therapist about such strategies.

Spotting and Heading Off Trouble

Another approach to managing difficult behavior is to learn the warning signs that indicate impending trouble and then distract the child, remove the child from the situation, or provide the child with other incompatible activities for the behavior. Some children show clear signs that they are becoming agitated, aggressive, or anxious. They do not explode out of the blue, but gradually escalate, first appearing worried or nervous, then muttering under their breath, then pacing and flapping their hands, and finally having a full-blown outburst complete with lashing out at others, destroying things, and being verbally abusive. A plan can be set up whereby the child is removed from the threatening situation and taken to a safe place. This might be a room in which he or she can pace, talk, or rant privately; a place with a couch to lie on while listening to soothing music; or a therapist or teacher who can guide the child through relaxation exercises (deep breathing, counting to 10, visualizing alternatives, and so on—see Chapter 8). It is important to engage in a proactive rather than a reactive way, lest a child be implicitly taught that acting out earns these potentially reinforcing activities.

Self-Monitoring and Reinforcing for Teens and Adults

Finally, some individuals with ASD, particularly adolescents and adults, can be taught to monitor their own behavior and reinforce themselves, thereby learning self-regulation and self-management techniques. Such systems are best set up by experienced clinicians. The essential ingredients are teaching the person to recognize the behavior that needs to be increased or decreased; training the person, often using videotapes, to reliably identify instances of occurrence or nonoccurrence of the behavior; and then regularly monitoring the behavior.

As an example, let's return to the interrupting behavior discussed above. A videotape of the child in the classroom could be made. Then the teacher or parent would sit down with the child and the videotape and point out when interrupting was occurring and when appropriate hand raising and other behaviors were present instead. The child would then be trained to reliably recognize the interrupting behavior. Once she was able to correctly say,

"Yes, I was interrupting there" or "No, that was not interrupting" about 80% of the time when watching the video, she would begin the self-monitoring phase. An index card would be taped to her desk; on it would be two columns, one labeled "Interrupting" and the other "Not interrupting." A watch with a soft alarm would be provided that would go off every few minutes. Whenever the alarm sounded, the child would have to place a check mark in one column or the other. By so doing, she would become increasingly aware of the interrupting behavior.

This recognition and monitoring of the behavior, in and of itself, is sometimes enough to alter the problem. Often several of the approaches described in this section need to be used in tandem. Changes need to be made in the environment, rules and rewards need to be set, alternative behaviors must be taught, and then the child can learn to monitor the behavior herself.

Consulting a Behavioral Specialist

While the best behavioral management plans seem like little more than "common sense" to many parents, it is often wise to create and monitor such plans with the help of a behavioral specialist trained in such techniques. Small oversights can unintentionally throw off the whole system. Children may be resistant to the plan parents try to set up, so it can be helpful to have a third party negotiate the terms of the "contract." Gradual fading of the reinforcement system can be difficult to manage, and assistance in determining the most appropriate pace at which to decrease the rewards is often helpful. Determining whether negative consequences should be added is best left to a professional. It is ideal if data are collected to indicate how successful the program is, when goals should be changed or added, and when new methods should be tried. With professional assistance, behavioral programs can be highly effective in changing some of the behaviors of people with ASD and alleviating much individual and family distress.

Medication

The use of medications to treat people with ASD has increased in recent years. Studies suggest that about half of all children with ASD in the United States have been prescribed a psycho-active medication, and that medication usage increases with age. Research studies have shown that levels of certain brain chemicals (neurotransmitters) are different in people with ASD, sometimes higher than they should be and sometimes lower. Although there are no medications that can reduce the primary symptoms of autism, such as difficulties in communication, appropriate use of medication can often increase the quality of life for both the child and the family. Medications can improve the child's ability to benefit from other forms of treatment and relieve significant distress for the affected person and those around her. For example, appropriate medical management of inattention and hyperactivity can help a child focus better at school and thus enhance the positive effects of the educational help provided. Similarly, easing social anxiety or reducing negative feelings about the self through medication can permit someone with ASD to participate in and benefit from a social skills group.

A wide range of medications have been used for ASD over the years. However, as yet no medication that reliably alters the core social and communication deficits of ASD in clinically meaningful ways has been found. The drugs that are commonly used with the ASD population address other symptoms and comorbid conditions, such as attention and activity level problems, depression, anxiety, aggression, repetitive thoughts or behaviors, sleep difficulties, tics, and seizures. The most commonly prescribed medications for those with ASD are stimulants such as Ritalin, Dexedrine, and Adderall; newer "atypical neuroleptics," such as Risperdal and Abilify; and selective serotonin reuptake inhibitors (SSRIs) such as Prozac, Zoloft, and Paxil. Note, however, that the evidence for the effectiveness of SSRIs for helping children with ASD is weak. These medications might help in individual cases, however.

The SSRIs are thought to work by increasing levels of the neurotransmitter serotonin in the brain, while stimulants and atypical neuroleptics act primarily on a different neurotransmitter, called dopamine, and block its function or decrease its level in the brain. Stimulants are the treatment of choice for attention and activity level problems and appear to work as well with children with ASD who have these disturbances as they do in children with attention deficit disorders alone. Risperdal and Abilify are medications first used for psychotic conditions, such as schizophrenia, but now found to be useful for the irritability, aggression, and explosive or unpredictable behavior sometimes seen in individuals with ASD. A study found that these types of medications are even more effective if they are combined with behavioral intervention to address behavioral challenges, such as tantrums and aggression.

How effective are these medications in treating ASD? To answer that question, we will digress a bit to explain the process by which we evaluate whether a therapy (any therapy—medical, behavioral, psychological) actually works. An obvious strategy would be to give people with ASD a medication and test them beforehand and afterward to see what the effect was. But more careful examination points out a few problems with this approach. Perhaps the symptoms would have gotten better on their own (for example, as the child got older) and the improvement had nothing to do with the drug. For this reason, therapy studies must use a *control sample*, which is a group of individuals very similar to those given the treatment—they must have the same diagnosis, the same level of functioning, be of similar ages, and so on—who differ only in not receiving the treatment.

It is well known among doctors that many patients improve after being given a medically neutral or inactive substance (a disguised sugar pill or harmless salt solution), called a *placebo*, if they believe that it has therapeutic powers. This improvement is known as the *placebo effect* and is thought to reflect the powers of hope and positive thinking as well as the more general effects of receiving attention from a doctor. So it is important that medications tried with your child have been shown to be more effective than a placebo. Previous studies have demonstrated that about one-third of people show clear improvement from a placebo. So we would want to know that a specific drug helps more than 30% of those who try it. Otherwise, why not spare the expense and potential side effects of the drug and just use the sugar pill? This can be tested in a research study in which the control group, rather than being untreated, is given a placebo instead.

The best studies include random assignment of individuals to the medication and placebo conditions and a lack of awareness on the parts of everyone involved in the study regarding which individuals are given which pill. Random assignment helps make sure that there are no consistent differences between the people getting placebo and those getting the medication that might account for differences in response. For example, if the first people to indicate interest in the study were assigned to the medication group, they might be more motivated to follow the requirements of the study or more hopeful of improvement, which could bias the results of the study. Conversely, if the first people to contact the researchers were those with the most severe symptoms and they were then assigned to the medication group, they might improve less because of their greater severity, again biasing the results. This is why assigning people to groups through a flip of a coin or other random procedure is so important. The second feature is that no one—not the parents, not the individual, and not even the doctor—knows who is getting the drug and who is receiving the placebo. This kind of investigation is called a *double-blind study* and again serves to minimize any biases that might be introduced (probably unintentionally) into the study.

Several double-blind, randomized studies have demonstrated that the atypical neuroleptics Risperdal and Abilify are indeed more helpful than placebo for people with ASD. They are the only two medications that have undergone enough testing to have been approved by the Food and Drug Administration (FDA) specifically for use in ASD. The results of studies of antidepressant use in ASD have been mixed, with some studies finding beneficial effects and others not, so at the time the second edition of this book was published, the FDA had not approved use of medications like Prozac specifically for ASD. This does not mean that your child's doctor might not wish to try a non-FDA-approved drug or that such a medication might not prove helpful for your child; it just means that more testing is needed before there would be widespread recommendation of this drug's use for individuals with ASD. Double-blind, placebo-controlled studies have found that many medications for attention-deficit/hyperactivity disorder (ADHD) help children with ASD who have additional problems with inattention and hyperactivity. None of these medications target the core symptoms of ASD, such as social difficulties or communication challenges, however. Typically, they address other problems, such as severe aggression, dysregulated behavior, or mood problems. This research is still in its infancy, and not enough studies have been done to be able to tell which individual characteristics predict the best success. For example, does the medication work best with a particular-age individual or with people with certain specific problems? And most medications carry some chance of side effects, so it is important to weigh risks, inconveniences, and financial costs carefully against the improvement that might be seen. Currently, double-blind, placebo-controlled, randomized studies suggest that medications can ease certain symptoms and thereby improve quality of life, but cannot alter the basic features of ASD. They are best used in combination with behavioral interventions.

Sensory Integration Therapy

Some children with ASD are overly sensitive to and easily overwhelmed by everyday sensations, such as certain sounds, tastes, textures, or smells, or by being touched. Their distress when encountering these sensations can be very intense. Parents sometimes describe the phenomenon as "sensory overload." One young woman said that when she was bombarded by unwanted sounds, smells, and sights, her body would "shut down." She described feeling completely detached, almost as if her body belonged to someone else or was a piece of furniture. One boy with ASD was so sensitive to smells that his mother called doctors in advance of his appointments to remind them not to wear perfume or scented antiperspirant. During one visit, he told his doctor pointedly that she had bad breath and threatened to leave unless she gargled with mouthwash. Many children with ASD find loud noises intolerable and will cover their ears when exposed to them. Some even have difficulty with noises that are not loud and don't bother others, such as the hum of an air conditioner or the sound of a baby crying. Other children have the opposite problem: they seem to crave certain sensations and will go out of their way (often inappropriately) to seek these sensations. For example, one young child diagnosed with ASD loved the texture of pantyhose. He could tell if a woman was wearing them from long distances and would do everything in his power to get near enough to feel them. A girl with autism loved to press her chin into the soft inner surface of people's elbows. Dr. Temple Grandin, the famed animal scientist with autism, craved the feeling of deep pressure; as a child, she would lie under couch cushions to create this sensation and later went on to develop her patented "squeeze machine" for the same purpose.

Sensory integration (SI) is the name of the process by which incoming sensations are interpreted, connected, and organized, something that is necessary for a child to feel safe and comfortable and able to function effectively in the environment. When a child is not able to make sense of sensory experiences, his or her behavior and learning may be profoundly affected, according to a theory advanced by Dr. Jean Ayres. She suggests that the unusual behaviors just described are due to sensory integrative dysfunction. Dr. Ayres noted that not only children with ASD, but also those with learning disabilities, cerebral palsy, and genetic syndromes, may suffer from sensory integrative dysfunction.

The goal of SI therapy is to decrease existing sensitivities, provide coping skills for remaining sensitivities, and increase tolerance for new sensations. This is done by exposing the child to a variety of sensory experiences through play and movement. The child is helped to explore many different materials and sensations. The child is given some control over the experiences in therapy but is also guided through certain activities, such as swinging, light brushing, or deep pressure, that are thought to promote better organization and interpretation of sensory input. A child who is very cautious, for example, might be guided gently through jumping activities, whereas a child who is wild and uncontained might learn to crawl through a tunnel of small chairs to learn more about spatial boundaries. Children usually enjoy the therapy, because the treatment setting is filled with fun things to climb and move on, such as ramps, platforms, mats, trapezes, and tubes. Sensory integration therapy is usually delivered by an occupational therapist. It is important to find a professional who has training in the underlying theory, as well as the specific techniques, of this treatment model.

Despite frequent anecdotal accounts from both professionals and parents that SI therapy can improve behavior and functioning, there hasn't been much research on the effectiveness of SI therapy. Although small randomized controlled trials have shown some positive effects of this type of therapy, more research is still needed. Nevertheless, many parents and children themselves report a calming effect with SI approaches. You may want to try them out, but as with all treatments reviewed here and especially those for which there is little research support, carefully assess the benefits you see. Do others, especially those unaware of the treatment, notice any changes in your child's behavior? Are any benefits you notice above and beyond those your child might show following a good night of sleep or participation in some other preferred or calming activity (like watching a favorite video)? You may find it helpful to keep a chart of your child's behavior, something as simple as two columns on a piece of paper for each day, one containing information about sleep, diet, therapy, and special circumstances and the other containing information about your child's behavior that day. In this way, you can keep track of any major changes and then examine their association with events in your child's life, including therapy. As always, financial cost introduces some limits. It is not possible to access every type of therapy for your child, nor desirable (from a time perspective) to do so. You will need to pick and choose among interventions and so be particularly careful in scrutinizing therapies whose effectiveness has yet to be established.

There are things other than SI therapy that may be useful in building your child's ability to organize and integrate experiences and body sensations. Movement and dance classes stress similar skills outside a therapeutic environment, as do individual sports and other fitness activities, such as martial arts training. You may want to consider some of these options as well.

Individual Psychotherapy

Traditional psychotherapy may help a limited number of individuals with ASD. Generally, individual psychotherapy involves discussion of emotions and gaining insight into behavior patterns or interpersonal issues. Since most children, adolescents, and even adults with ASD have limited self-awareness, do not naturally make social comparisons, and often show little insight into the nature and reasons for their difficulties, this form of psychotherapy is often not very helpful for them. Additionally, the realm in which the majority of problems arise for those with ASD, social situations, are best dealt with in larger group formats, rather than in individual therapy sessions. One of the chief difficulties encountered in autism is the lack of automatic generalization, from one situation to another, from one interaction to another, from one setting to another, from one person to another. It is therefore unlikely that work done in a one-to-one setting with an understanding therapist will generalize to group social situations involving peers. Thus, group therapy (often in the form of social skills training) may be a better way to address the specific issues inherent in ASD.

Under some circumstances, however, individual psychotherapy may be warranted, especially for the highest-functioning adolescents and adults, who have gained some ability to understand their own and others' emotional states and behaviors. Individual psychotherapy may, in these limited circumstances, be helpful in dealing with the anxiety, depression, and emotional dysregulation that often accompany ASD and the pain that may accompany the growing awareness of their differences from others. Counseling should still be highly structured and rather more directive and concrete than typical psychotherapy with individuals who don't have ASD. There should be a clear focus on specific problems, developing more effective methods to cope with them, and planning strategies to maximize the person's potential and help him attain important life skills such as job-related social behaviors. The therapy may be highly directive and may even involve "field trips" into the community to encourage development of specific independent functioning skills (riding the bus, interviewing for a job, ordering food in a restaurant, and the like). Studies have shown that cognitive-behavioral therapy, which focuses on understanding one's thoughts and how they influence behavior, is effective for addressing anxiety symptoms in high-functioning adolescents and adults with ASD. We talk more about cognitive-behavioral therapy in Chapter 8, and additional information is included in the Resources.

Dietary Treatments

Some professionals have advocated the use of special diets, vitamin supplements, or both to manage some symptoms associated with ASD. In recent years, a theory has been formed that some cases of autism are caused by food allergies, specifically severe allergic reactions to gluten, a protein found in flour, and casein, a protein found in milk products, that irritate or damage the brain and lead to the unusual behaviors associated with ASD. So far this hypothesis is based on clinical observations and parent reports rather than well-controlled scientific studies. It is clear, however, that many children with ASD do have difficulties with their gastrointestinal systems, and this may result in problems such as reflux, constipation, and diarrhea. It is important to talk with your pediatrician, and if need be, a gastroenterologist if your child is having these symptoms. Feeding issues, such as picky eating, are also very common. Again, your pediatrician should be able to discuss strategies for helping with these issues.

As with understanding the potential risks and benefits associated with medications, future research investigations on dietary interventions are very much needed. Some parents report improvement of their child's behavior when certain products are removed from their diet. When children are undergoing elimination diets (that is, diets that systematically remove one type of food at a time), it is not possible to have parents and children themselves be "blind" to what group they are in. However, it is perfectly possible to randomly assign children to diet or no-diet groups and to have the scientists evaluating the children be unaware of group assignment. This needs to be done before the effectiveness of these therapies can be known. It is always recommended that such diets be conducted in collaboration with a dietician or other medical professional who is knowledgeable about potential side effects or risks and can ensure that proper nutritional needs are met.

Another form of dietary treatment for ASD is vitamin supplements. Dr. Bernard Rimland, who was one of the first professionals to propose a biological cause for autism, was a supporter of so-called megavitamin therapy, which involves administering large doses (much larger than in a typical vitamin supplement) of vitamin B_6 and magnesium. These two vitamins are usually given in combination, because the mineral magnesium is necessary for proper absorption of vitamin B_6. Dimethylglycine, or DMG, is another "natural substance" found in many health food stores reported to help autistic symptoms. Many parents report improvement in a wide variety of behaviors, including eye contact, social initiation, language, mood, and aggression, when their children are taking these supplements. A few studies have been conducted, some using double-blind or placebo-controlled methods, but the evidence of effectiveness is mixed. Almost all the studies had some significant limitations, such as examining very small numbers of children, not randomly assigning subjects to groups, or not using standardized methods of assessing change. We always recommend that megavitamin therapy be conducted with the collaboration of an experienced physician, because side effects of the vitamin treatments are possible, and doctors are not yet sure that the very high doses typically used are not toxic in some way.

Family Support

A final realm of treatment is the family. Relieving family distress should by no means be considered secondary or unimportant, although this topic falls at the end of this chapter. Many of the preceding treatments, if they are effective and help your child, will by extension help you and your family in general. To the extent that significant difficulties remain for members of the family, however, additional support may be necessary. Most urban areas have support or self-help groups for parents and families of people with ASD. In some areas, there are even regular meetings that are specifically for families of higher-functioning children, so that the topics of focus are specifically relevant for those with milder or higher-functioning symptoms. If such meetings are not available in your area, don't despair, because most support groups will still make a strong effort to have some of their meetings centered on higher-functioning individuals. You just may need to call ahead and get a schedule of topics to know when it will be most relevant for you to attend. Parents often find it useful to talk with other parents, who understand better than professionals what you are going through and who may have useful remedies for situations you find your family in, even if their children are functioning at different levels. These support groups do indeed make it clear that you are not alone. Feelings of isolation at the time of diagnosis are almost universal among parents. Joining a support group will diminish those feelings considerably, as well as provide much constructive and practical assistance. Whether or not you attend regular meetings of such support groups, do contact your state autism society, an invaluable resource for relevant community programs, books, conferences, and Internet sites.

You should also contact the government agency in your state that provides services to people with disabilities. There is usually a long eligibility process that takes into account the severity of symptoms, your child's functioning level and age, your family's resources (financial and otherwise), and the impact your child is having on your family system. If your child is found to be eligible under your state's rules, you may receive funding for a variety of different services (vocational training, residential care, preschool programs). Respite care is a service that provides trained paraprofessionals who can take care of your child for short periods of time, giving you and your family some needed time off. At its best, respite care is much the same as having a highly trained and trustworthy babysitter who is free. As your child gets older, your state agency for people with disabilities may also be able to provide vocational assistance, both in training your child for employment and in helping him find and keep a job. Additionally, there are a variety of assisted or semi-independent living situations that may be useful as your child ages into adulthood and you or the child desire new and more autonomous residential arrangements. We have more to say on this topic in Chapter 9.

Family and marital therapy can also be useful, especially if your family is experiencing significant stress related to the raising of your child. Parents may have significant anxiety or depression about their child's diagnosis or future, irrational guilt about having in some way caused the problem, anger and frustration about the availability of services, resentment about the effects of a difficult child on the family, and so forth. A skilled family or marital therapist can help you work through these feelings, learn to cope with the needs of your child, and still maintain some semblance of a life. If there are significant disagreements about discipline, other parenting issues, or treatment, a family therapist can be invaluable in constructively and adaptively addressing them, helping sort out the different choices, and disentangling personal or marital issues from the needs of your child with ASD.

Parents as Treatment Managers

One of your biggest challenges as parents of a child with ASD is bringing all the therapy options together into a cohesive treatment program that addresses your child's needs and promotes development in an integrated fashion. Your child may work on improving her social skills in an outpatient therapy group in a clinic, at school, at home, and in speech–language therapy. It is necessary that someone coordinate the different goals of each of these interventions, taking care that all involved are working toward a common set of needs and not at cross-purposes. Often this role falls to you.

Besides this day-to-day management, you will need to be aware of the changes in your child's and your family's needs over time. No treatment plan will be adequate forever. Some challenges will diminish with time and intervention; others may emerge as new developmental stages are reached and the skills needed to negotiate them change. It may be necessary to have your child reevaluated every few years by a professional who has expertise in ASD and knows your child well to be sure that the treatment "package" continues to be useful.

The most difficult challenge of all, though, may be deciding which treatments to pursue in the first place. Most parents feel acute pressure to find the best treatment for their child. Often this quest involves trying emerging interventions that appear to show promise but have not yet been thoroughly researched. For some parents, the need to leave no stone unturned, to try *anything* that might be helpful, outweighs the potential risks and financial costs involved. But few of the interventions available, including some of the ones discussed in this chapter, have been studied adequately. And you can count on hearing about newly developed ones for which extreme claims of effectiveness are made. Typically, these interventions will not have been subjected to the kind of experimental research that provides information about what type of child benefits from the treatment, what particular symptoms of autism the treatment addresses, through what mechanism the intervention creates the changes it claims to make, and what "dose" of the therapy is required. You will have to ask the tough questions to determine the risk–benefit ratio of trying any such new therapy. For what age child does this treatment seem to work best? Does the child need to have language to benefit from the intervention? If so, how much? What kind of assessment is carried out before and after the treatment to determine the gains made? Be particularly suspicious of any treatment that claims to work equally well for all children with ASD.

It may be even more helpful to talk with a professional who is familiar with ASD and the long history of its treatment before choosing new treatments for your child. Hearing about earlier "miracle cures" that turned out, once researched, to be ineffective may give you a different, wiser perspective. In the early 2000s, the digestive hormone secretin was touted as a miraculous "cure" for autism and received much attention on national news programs. Many children received intravenous infusions of secretin, without any evidence that it was effective other than the anecdotal media accounts. No evaluation of children before and after secretin treatment had been carried out to document the claims. After this frenzy, multiple separate studies involving hundreds of children nationwide demonstrated definitively that children with ASD show no more benefit from secretin than they do from intravenous infusions of saline (salt water, a placebo that has no therapeutic potential). Secretin remains one of the most well-studied interventions for ASD. Although it has been debunked, the fervor it inspired demonstrates how acquiring information from the wrong sources can mislead families and misdirect resources.

At the least, ineffective treatments are costly and delay the provision of effective treatments; in the worst-case scenarios, they may actually be harmful to your child. So be sure that all your questions are answered by someone you feel comfortable with and who has experience and expertise in the autism field. Be sure to check out local facilities and treatment programs, which are unlikely to have received media attention but may well be based on sound educational and therapeutic practices.

Part II

LIVING WITH HIGH-FUNCTIONING AUTISM SPECTRUM DISORDER

5

Channeling Your Child's Strengths

A GUIDING PRINCIPLE

Barbara and Jose held hands as they drove home from Alberto's school, where their son was enrolled in first grade. Alberto had been diagnosed with ASD during the summer, and now his teacher was reporting that he was having a very difficult time with both peers and adults in school. He wasn't interested in playing with the other children, and he often refused to follow the rules. Despite being very intelligent, he rarely did his work, preferring to draw pictures of his favorite computer game characters. If this pattern continued, he might not be promoted to second grade.

As the car pulled into the driveway, Alberto raced from the house in his stocking feet to embrace his parents and tell them about his most recent achievement in his favorite computer game. Jose looked at his son's smiling face, felt the tenderness in his hug, and experienced the now-familiar pain of knowing that others couldn't see how truly wonderful his child was. How could he and Barbara help their son take his enthusiasm and passion to school with him? How could they teach Alberto to apply the skills that had made him a neighborhood legend at computer games to math, classroom rules, and friends?

Janice smiled with delight as she opened the wrinkled paper bag that 12-year-old Sameer had just handed her. Sameer rarely commented on her likes and dislikes or on their interactions during their therapy sessions, but obviously he had noticed the type of pen she used, remembered the single occasion she had mentioned her music tastes, and registered which snacks she occasionally left sitting on her desk. There in the bag, which he had taped closed and labeled "JA" in black marker, were her favorite model of pen, filled with ink in her favorite color; a bag of her favorite type of potato chip; and a home-made CD containing her favorite song—recorded 50 times. Sameer's naturally prodigious memory had helped him show Janice how important their relationship was to him, and Janice could see from his beaming face as she thanked him that this was a hugely satisfying accomplishment for this boy with high-functioning ASD.

For children like Alberto and Sameer, everyday activities are often a big challenge. Normal, routine interactions with others can seem so difficult. As parents, you can see your child's admirable, endearing qualities, but all too often the world seems blind to them. And because you spend a lot of time and energy helping your child meet the demands of the outside world, you too can end up focusing largely on your child's deficits and differences. This chapter offers you the opportunity to adopt a new mind-set, to begin thinking of your child's strengths first and his weaknesses second whenever you want to help him navigate the waters of a world that can be difficult to understand. Chapters 6 through 9 offer a long list of specific strategies for helping your child succeed and enjoy life at home, at school, in the social arena, and, as the child matures, in the workplace and other adult settings. What underlies them all, however, is the simple principle that you can channel your child's unusual behaviors and ways of thinking into positive achievements.

Recognizing and capitalizing on your child's strengths, and helping others to do so too, can go a long way toward making up for his or her areas of difficulty. We've found, in fact, that asking yourself how you can take advantage of the true gifts associated with ASD, or how you can creatively use the unique ways of thinking or behaving associated with ASD, tends to produce many more solutions than strategies that concentrate on addressing your high-functioning child's weaknesses. By consistently calling attention to your child's ability to adapt in unique ways, you help others see your child's admirable qualities and also cement the positive bonds between parent and child. Perhaps most important, you help build your child's self-esteem. Success breeds success, and children with ASD who are given opportunities to succeed tend to adapt to the non-ASD world more quickly and completely than those who are taught to view life as one problem after another.

In Part I of this book we discussed how and why children with high-functioning ASD are different from typical children and what we do to try to overcome their problems. There is no question that trying to reduce the severity of disability is an important aspect of treatment. Some children with ASD are able to change and improve to a significant degree. But we urge all parents not to stop there. You can tweak the environment too, in effect making it adapt to what your child has to offer. This is what living with ASD is all about, and it is the guiding principle behind all the suggestions we make in the chapters to come.

This chapter describes six strengths commonly seen in children with high-functioning ASD and provides ideas for how to use them to help your child on a daily basis. You'll see them incorporated into our suggestions for living with ASD at home, at school, with friends, in jobs, and in adult life in the following chapters, and we hope you'll focus on them whenever you have to come up with creative solutions on your own.

Enough research has been conducted on long-term outcome to know that children with ASD can live fruitful and happy lives. Dr. Temple Grandin, the extremely successful animal scientist with ASD introduced earlier in the book, describes her achievements by stating, "I developed my talent area. Often, we put too much emphasis on the disabled area. You have to focus on the skills you are good at and figure out how to use them to work around your disability." Children who begin early to capitalize on their strengths are laying an important foundation for future success.

Inez is a 35-year-old woman with ASD. Every weekday she takes the bus to the campus of the university in her town and passes through the impressive, vaulted entrance of the campus library. She spends the day working in the archives department, locating old articles for students and organizing the library's collection. Inez has always been passionate about history, and this job gives her an opportunity to earn a living while keeping close to her intense interests. Her boss says she is the most efficient employee he has ever had, describing her knowledge of the university's archival collection as "remarkable."

Inez may never have gotten where she is today without the help of her parents. They realized that her interest in history, which often interfered with other aspects of her education, was not going to disappear and was an integral part of who she was. They resolved to stimulate, rather than discourage, her passion for history and make it applicable to the "real world" and future careers whenever they saw the potential to do so. In high school, they successfully lobbied her teachers to incorporate history into every class and many assignments. In this way, Inez broadened her focus a bit, learning not just about world history, but also about the history of science, the history of computers, and the history and evolution of different languages. They enrolled Inez in a history club, where she met adults with history-related careers (such as genealogy). Her parents even read some of the same books Inez was devouring so that they could chat about history at dinner each evening. When a job counselor mentioned the library archivist position to them, they recognized at once that this was a great opportunity for Inez to apply her enthusiasm in a productive way. After speaking with Inez, who was ecstatic about the prospect of working in an archives department, her parents spoke with her potential employer about ASD and both its special strengths and its limitations. He was open-minded about the idea of employing Inez, and he hired her. Although it took some time and effort for her employer and her parents to teach Inez about the rules of the workplace, she has flourished in the position and was recently named "Employee of the Month" in her department.

Inez is a good example of how the unique behaviors and special interests associated with ASD, considered "symptoms" by the doctors who diagnosed your child, can instead be seen as "strengths" and can be used to help your child be successful in life. The six characteristics discussed in this chapter fall into two groups: *true strengths*, abilities that are beneficial in and of themselves; and *unique behaviors* that can be channeled into strengths with a little creativity and a shift of perspective. Your child is unlikely to demonstrate every strength we discuss or to be able to channel all unique behaviors into strengths, but through observation you should be able to determine which ones your own child possesses and which strategies will be most successful for him or her.

True Strengths and Natural Abilities

Many people with ASD demonstrate a remarkable capacity for memorization, superior academic skills (particularly in reading and spelling), and/or strong visualization skills. These skills are valuable to school success and future career potential. Whether you have ASD or not, it is useful to have a good memory, good reading and spelling skills, and highly developed visual–spatial abilities. Which can you see in your child?

Remarkable Memory

Other people often marvel at the remarkable memories, particularly for details and facts, of those with ASD. In some cases, this memory can seem "photographic," enabling perfect recollection after only a single or brief exposure to the information. Other times, it is the sheer volume and precision of the memory that is so impressive.

Eight-year-old Robert recently astounded guests at his parents' dinner party when he told them, "The standard spacing of railroad tracks in the United States is based on the original spacing of wheels on an imperial Roman war chariot, which was 4 feet and 8 and one-half inches." Fascinated by the Greco-Roman War, Robert spent much of his free time devouring books on the subject rather than playing outside with the neighborhood kids and often regaled his parents at the dinner table with perfectly recalled details about what he had read. As his parents recognized his superior memory capacity, they encouraged him to use this skill in a functional manner whenever possible. They gave him a list of topics that other kids liked to talk about (the local professional basketball team, computer games, and so on), which he committed to memory and then used to converse more appropriately with his peers. They entered him in the town spelling bee, in which he placed second. And they encouraged his teachers to begin working on his multiplication tables, which he mastered in a matter of weeks. His parents were pleasantly surprised to find that Robert's prodigious memory was not limited to Greco-Roman War facts, but was in fact usable in a variety of other domains.

Superior Academic Skills

Besides having strong memories for facts and other information, many children with ASD have stronger than average academic abilities, typically in one or two specific domains. Advanced vocabulary is one example. Learning and using new or sophisticated words comes easily to some children with ASD, as we've seen in many examples throughout this book. Spelling is another common strength. And many children with ASD can sound out words far beyond their own grade level (although their actual understanding of what they are reading may be more consistent with their grade level or even lower).

One way to use this strength is to have your child tutor less capable peers in school. This can carry over to areas that may be more difficult for your child, such as social interaction, while also improving your child's self-esteem and potentially increasing interest in peers.

Norma had a hard time interacting with the other students in her sixth-grade class. They often teased her, and she frequently thought their interests were silly. However, she was an excellent student, particularly in English. She could sound out and spell any word, even those at the college level. The school psychologist suggested to her teacher that asking Norma to tutor kids who didn't read very well might be a good way to increase her self-esteem. Norma greatly enjoyed her work as a peer tutor. It not only showcased her talents and helped her feel valued by her peers, but also allowed her to connect socially in a predictable, structured, and comfortable way.

Visual Thinking

Many people with ASD are what we call "visual thinkers," which gives them advanced skills in things like completing puzzles, reading maps, or quickly learning the layout of a building. In her book

Thinking in Pictures, Dr. Temple Grandin describes translating words automatically into pictures. When someone speaks to her, their words are instantly transformed into a series of images that tell a visual story. She describes her thoughts as visual representations, rather than as the stream of words that make up thoughts for most verbal thinkers.

Much of our world was created *by* verbal thinkers *for* verbal thinkers. News programs and newspapers are in words. Instruction manuals usually rely on words, as do job listings. People communicate and interact predominantly with words. This can present some obstacles for people whose minds use a visually based system of thinking, but it also opens up possibilities to excel in ways difficult or impossible for verbal thinkers. Dr. Grandin, for example, describes how she can "test" cow-handling facilities by "operating them" in her mind, actually giving herself a "cow's-eye view" and experiencing firsthand what a cow would see walking through the facility. Verbal thinkers might be able to talk themselves through this type of experience, but they would miss important details.

By no means does everyone with strong visualization skills have ASD. Most artists, graphic designers, illustrators, architects, mathematicians, and engineers are visual thinkers. This style is simply a different way of processing information, not a deficit, and it opens up potential career niches not available to most verbal thinkers.

Ronnie, a college student with high-functioning ASD, had known for a long time that he was a visual thinker. He had been using his visualization abilities to bolster his performance in school for most of his life. However, he never realized how much of an advantage visual thinking could be until he began the study of architecture. On his first project, he was surprised that many of his classmates were unable to detect design flaws until they constructed a mock-up model of the structure. Ronnie was able to think of a design and examine it closely in his mind. He could visualize the way it would look from different angles and the difficulties it might present for people using the space. He found that by the time he created a mock-up he had already worked out a viable design. This strength also helped him make social contacts. As his classmates became aware of his natural ability, many approached Ronnie to ask for his evaluation of their work.

You can also use your child's visual thinking style to teach concepts, explain rules, organize activities, or anticipate changes in routine. For example, the use of visual graphics or objects rather than verbal explanations or word problems may help your child grasp mathematical concepts more quickly. A fun way to practice math with your child is to use chocolate chips in addition or subtraction problems, allowing them to be eaten when your child provides a correct answer. The same principle could be used with pennies: you can allow your child to keep the pennies earned for correct solutions. Allowing your child to illustrate her work or to find pictures related to the topic she is writing about may enhance her motivation and learning.

For a visual thinker, pictures of things to be done along with pictures of the positive consequences for completing these tasks can be a strong motivator. An example of this system was provided in Chapter 4.

Annie's mother dreaded the daily struggle over homework. Every evening Annie protested doing her assignments because she preferred to sit and draw pictures. When her mother tried to talk to Annie about this issue, it seemed to "go in one ear and out the other." Considering Annie's strength in visualization (as evidenced by her superb drawing skills), her mother decided to ask Annie to help her make a pictorial after-school schedule: snack, homework, video, bedtime. Annie enjoyed making the schedule and seemed less resistant to follow it now that she understood what was expected and took ownership of developing it. If she completed all the items on the schedule on time, she could draw a star on a chart that accompanied the schedule. At the end of each week, five stars would be redeemable for a trip to the art supplies store to purchase a new marker or drawing pad. The visual reminder helped Annie remain aware that doing her homework each night would earn her the right to watch a video before bedtime. It also provided her with a long-range goal to help her maintain motivation throughout the week. Although Annie still preferred drawing to math, the adoption of a visual reminder system drastically cut down on the need for Annie's mother to nag and fight with her over homework.

Unique Behaviors That Can Become Strengths

There are other characteristics associated with high-functioning ASD that can similarly be used to your child's advantage. Sadly, however, you may be more used to hearing these positive character-istics identified as deficits. Problems that children with ASD have in school and the social world are often related to their inflexibil-ity, single-mindedness, and difficulty relating to peers. But there's another way to look at—and capitalize on—these behaviors and ways of thinking. With a little creativity and thoughtfulness, these too can become strengths.

Recognizing Order and Following Rules

People with ASD often navigate the world by forming explicit "rules" or recognizing patterns about how things work, the ways people interact, and how events typically unfold. Parents are often amazed by their child's ability to analyze information and extract a set of patterns or rules by which something operates. One ado-lescent girl with ASD commented that she noticed that one of the authors (G. D.) preferred clothing with horizontal stripes, whereas a coworker preferred clothing with vertical stripes. In fact, neither of us had consciously noticed that we had this preference, but when we mentally reviewed our wardrobes we had to admit that she was right. While we don't know exactly what facility enables people with ASD to see certain patterns in behavior and conduct, we do know that this ability can compensate for the lack of natural intuition about social situations associated with ASD. Rules, patterns, laws, and principles can help a person who doesn't have great "common sense" about how to behave in certain situations feel comfortable and more sure of the appropriate course of action.

Hariko is a young adult with ASD who graduated from college and works as a medical transcriptionist in a hospital. In explaining her success, she divulged her "secret" of closely watching others to formulate rules of social behavior. Even when she was a child, she noted, she had observed peers for clues about appropriate conduct or comments. "I watched what they did or said in a certain situation and then memorized that rule in case it ever happened to me. And I was always so happy when someone would just *tell* me the rule! I remember being so relieved when my mother said that I should look at someone and give a wave if they said 'Hi' to me in the hall," Hariko explained.

The same tendency can lead many children with ASD to enthusiastically embrace existing rules and become great law-abiding citizens. The rules must, however, be clear, explicit, and consistent, or the child with ASD is likely to challenge their logic—possibly relentlessly. Alberto, for example, couldn't help questioning why he and his classmates should be limited to walking in the hallways when running would get them where they were supposed to be faster. And why on earth should they share a toy with a peer when they were still having fun playing with it? To a child with ASD, these communal rules and social niceties may seem arbitrary and counterintuitive unless the logic behind them is clearly explained.

The desire for rules and order can be used to enlist your child's help with chores around the home. Taking on household responsibilities can be difficult for all children, but if you match the task to your child's natural inclinations, it can be much easier.

Terrell loved things to be in the "correct" place. As a young child, he would become very upset if the salt and pepper shakers were not placed in the middle of the kitchen table, neatly centered on a doily. As a teenager, he spent hours elaborately arranging his collections of rocks and bottle tops in categories according to rules his parents could never quite discern. Since he was so orderly, his parents thought he might be very good at mowing the lawn, but Terrell hated the noise of the lawnmower and got very frustrated because the blades of grass didn't appear to be cut evenly. Instead, his parents asked him to help them clean their home office and organize their files. Once they generated the appropriate filing system, Terrell undertook this task with gusto and performed as well as the best secretary. He later got a job at a local secondhand store, where he organized donated items by category for resale.

You can also use your child's inclination to follow rules to increase his social opportunities. Children with ASD are likely to find social interactions that occur in rule-governed contexts more comfortable. A great example of social interaction in a rule-governed context is playing board games. Many board games not only follow a predictable routine but rely on other strengths associated with ASD, such as memory and visual thinking. Other examples include trivia games, spelling or word construction games, card games, and chess.

Passion and Conviction

Parents of children with ASD often lament their child's single-mindedness about certain subjects or interests—usually to the detriment of necessities such as schoolwork, chores, and personal hygiene. But the very same tendency for focus makes these children diligent students of the subjects that intrigue them and very high achievers in those areas.

Neela was diagnosed with ASD in preschool after her parents noticed she was exhibiting tendencies similar to those of her older brother with ASD. One of Neela's special interests was computer games, which she enjoyed so much that she taught herself how to program her own games, earning her high status among kids in her neighborhood and at school. In junior high, she started a business making personalized screensavers for her parents' friends, earning her some much-desired pocket money. In her sophomore year of high school, Neela volunteered in the computer science department of the large state university in her city, where she distinguished herself so much that she was offered a paying job the next summer. Neela is now enrolled at the Massachusetts Institute of Technology (MIT), an accomplishment her parents never could have dreamed of when she was an isolated preschooler who spent much of her time reciting dialogue from Disney videos.

Gene, who also has ASD, is only in high school, but he's so passionate about chemistry that he's enrolled in college-level courses, where he excels and is a favored participant in class discussions. His professor was amazed at Gene's knowledge of the basic chemical compounds that make up everyday items, like cleanser and antiperspirant, information that he frequently shared with the class. The professor only became aware of Gene's diagnosis after the semester ended and Gene mentioned it in passing. To Gene's professor, his knowledge was highly valued and practical, not a symptom of a disorder.

The same zeal for specific interests seems to instill in people with ASD a strong conviction in their own beliefs. They can be virtually unwavering in the face of opposing ideas or arguments.

Laney was fascinated by recycling and the science of conservation. In her free time, she studied ways to reduce waste and increase use of recycled materials. When she first approached her junior high school principal about her ideas, he didn't really pay attention. But after she talked extensively with several teachers and paid a few more visits to the principal's office, he implemented some of the changes Laney had suggested. Her dedication and her passion had overcome the lack of interest of those around her and contributed to community improvement.

Whenever possible, incorporate your child's interests into school-related activities. By doing this often and broadly, you will maximize the likelihood that these interests will someday be channeled in a functional way that leads to a job or a career. For example, reading lessons might focus on topics that intrigue your child. English or writing assignments might be adapted to allow your child to write about her area of interest. Math word problems that incorporate the child's special interest can be devised. Catalogs of favored items (for example, sprinkler system parts) or menus from favorite restaurants can be used to teach your child money concepts. In social studies, your child can construct a timeline of important discoveries in the domain of her interest (for example, animals, computers, geography). Other examples of how to use special interests to motivate your child in the classroom are given in Chapter 7. How to find a good match between your child's interests and the workplace will be discussed in Chapter 9.

You can also use your child's special interest in a topic as a reward for completing chores, homework, or any other less preferred routine. An old adage of learning theory is "something of value should never be given freely." In other words, recognize what is reinforcing for and desirable to your child and make him work a bit for access to it. For example, allow your child to watch his favorite train video or read his plumbing fixtures catalog only *after* he's brushed his teeth and put on his pajamas. If your child loves using the computer, at school the teacher might make computer time contingent upon finishing a certain number of math problems. But some caution needs to be exercised in restricting your child's access to his or her favorite topics or activities. It is very important to make goals realistic and rewards frequent. For some children, like Annie, who preferred drawing to doing her homework, making the reward contingent upon completion of a week's worth of homework might be sufficient. For younger children and those with a shorter attention span (or a greater dislike of the task at hand), rewards should be more frequent. It is easier to start with more frequent rewards and space them out as your child adjusts to the idea of working for access to his favorite items or activities.

Another way to use your child's zeal for a topic in a functional way is to find peers who share the interest. This can create new opportunities for social interaction and practicing peer relationship skills.

When Thomas, a teen with ASD, was introduced to John, a typically developing boy a few years younger, the two hit it off immediately because both were fascinated by principles of engineering and their applications to environmental problems. The boys spent time together drawing up elaborate designs for machinery that would "save the world," and a genuine friendship blossomed. Because he enjoyed having an audience for his ideas, Thomas learned to become more flexible and less controlling in his interactions with John and thus avoided many of the pitfalls that had plagued his previous social relationships.

One of the best ways to find peers with common interests is to locate clubs or groups devoted to those interests. A child with ASD who has expertise in astronomy or space travel might thrive in a science fiction club or a fan club for television shows dealing with the subject matter. In these settings, a well-developed memory and possession of a great store of knowledge about a particular topic is an asset and can earn social status. One child who took great interest in a fantasy-based card game had little desire to socially engage his classmates, and, in fact, this interest frequently interfered with his social interactions. On weekends, however, he looked forward to attending tournaments and playing against and interacting with other children who shared his interest. He described these tournaments as the only time he felt he "really fit in." Another child, who was an avid reader, started his own book club. By having a prearranged topic of discussion, this group helped the child prepare for social interactions and provided him with assurance that he would know what to talk about. More on how to use your child's passionate interests in social situations appears in Chapter 8.

Comfort and Compatibility with Adults

Children with ASD often have difficulty getting along with their peers, whose behavior they may find unpredictable or capricious. Adults are usually more consistent and more accommodating than peers, so many youngsters with ASD prefer the company of adults. The fact that children with ASD are sophisticated in their language use and interests makes adults enjoy their company as well.

Johan fastened his top button and smoothed down his hair. He smiled with excitement as he walked downstairs to meet his parents' friends who were coming over for dinner. Johan loved to talk to people, but he had difficulty interacting with the children at school. They often made jokes that were confusing to him, and sometimes they made fun of his conversation topics. But he always had a great time interacting with his parents' adult friends. They talked about more interesting things and they never made fun of him. His parents had noted this preference when he was younger, so they invited their friends over more often and encouraged Johan to participate. They found that even though these positive social interactions weren't with peers, each occasion seemed to increase Johan's comfort and interest in just being around others, both adults *and* children. His parents were delighted that his comfort with adults had translated into success with peers during a recent class trip to a nursing home. When students were asked to mingle with the elderly residents, many felt shy or uncertain about what to do. Johan didn't hesitate to introduce himself to the adults. The residents found him charming and were pleased to have his attention. Johan's classmates were astounded by the contrast with the hesitancy he showed during interactions with them. They saw a new side of Johan, and for the remainder of the visit many tagged along with him so that his adeptness with adults could cover for their own discomfort.

Identifying Your Child's Strengths

The six characteristics listed above are a good place to start in identifying your own child's potential strengths. But keep in mind that it's not always easy or simple to identify strengths. Nor is it easy to determine which behaviors that usually manifest themselves as weaknesses can be redirected to make them strengths. When your child's endless discussion of the detailed features of myriad video game characters is getting in the way of social interactions and family plans, it can be a challenge to recognize that this behavior is reflective of a great memory. Observe your child's behavior in a variety of contexts and consider the following questions:

• *What does your child enjoy?* When she has free time, what does she choose to do? What things does she ask you about? What things does she tell you about? What kinds of items does she ask you to buy? What subjects in school does your child enjoy the most? In what types of family activities does she have the most fun?

- *When is your child most successful?* Think about areas in which your child is currently doing well or has succeeded in the past. Are there particular subjects in school in which your child gets good grades? Does your child do well at spelling bees or memorizing math facts but have trouble doing word problems or answering questions about what he's read? Does your child perform better in certain types of social settings than in others? Can he join a group of kids playing a board game, but not ride bikes with the neighborhood kids? Do adults often comment on how charming your child is and appear puzzled at his difficulties with peers?

- *What does your child not mind doing?* Also considering what your child least dislikes can be informative. Does your child willingly go to the dictionary to look up a word for you when you're reading the newspaper, but asks you to do the simplest arithmetic for her, such as "How many days are left in this month?" A child might refuse to help with mowing the lawn but not mind organizing the bric-a-brac in the living room or putting away the dishes.

It may be helpful to record your observations in a journal. Nothing elaborate is needed, simply a daily or weekly list of things that your child seemed to enjoy, tolerate, or succeed at and the settings in which the activities took place. Ask your child's teachers or care providers about the activities your child enjoys and excels in during class or after-school care. Compare the answers you get from others to your own ideas to obtain a broader picture of your child's behavior. See if a consistent picture emerges.

Depending on his age and abilities, your child may be able to participate in the process of identifying strengths. An open discussion with your child about his unique characteristics can build self-esteem (some additional resources for doing this informal interview are mentioned at the end of Chapter 8). One psychologist who frequently works with children with ASD frames the task as creating an "operating manual" for the child. Explain to your child that you have decided to create such a manual to help the child better understand himself and to help others better understand him. Make a list of things you have noticed your child enjoys and excels at. Ask if your child agrees with these strengths and if he can think of any others. If he needs help, give some examples of possible strengths ("Are you good at reading?"; "Do you like everything neat and in the right place?"; "Can you tell if I'm going the wrong way to school?").

Finally, examine the observations you have made and look for patterns or themes. Use the list of strengths that we described as a guideline, but be open to other possibilities. Do the areas in which you've seen your child succeed have anything in common? Are there shared features in the types of activities your child prefers? During what kinds of activities does your child have the most fun? Do the things your child enjoys or is willing to do reflect strong memory, academic or visual skills, a desire for order and rules, passion for a topic, or a gravitation toward adult company?

Remember that every child is unique and that your child may show different strengths than the most common ones described in this chapter. Perhaps your daughter's verbal skills are extremely advanced, suggesting that explaining something verbally would work better than making a visual list for her. Maybe your son craves quiet and displays a calm, gentle nature that would make him an ideal candidate for a job working with animals. Be open to all possibilities. The main idea is to look for themes and commonalities among your child's preferences, inclinations, strengths, and passions and then to use them on a daily basis to inform all sorts of issues, from chores, discipline, and positive family relationships, to school and future jobs.

There are many practical reasons to take advantage of the unique abilities that are part and parcel of ASD. Taking advantage of your child's natural abilities can make things easier for both you and your child. But again, the most important aspect of focusing on strengths may be the boost it can provide to your child's self-esteem. Many children with ASD are painfully aware of their shortcomings. They work overtime at school, at home, and with therapists to try to overcome their difficulties. Often those who interact with these special and unique children fail to emphasize the many areas in which they excel. Capitalizing on the things your child does well can help you feel good about yourself and your child. For your child, maintaining a focus on strengths and natural abilities can have long-term positive effects on motivation, self-esteem, and achievement. In the remaining chapters of this book, we give specific guidelines for how to use your child's strengths to overcome the difficulties often associated with ASD that arise at home, in school, in the workplace, and with others.

6

High-Functioning Autism Spectrum Disorder at Home

Parenting a child with ASD can be a challenging role. You already spend a lot of time and energy managing your child's treatment, coordinating your child's education, and serving as social coach in your child's friendships and extended-family relationships. At home, things should be easier. Often, however, they are not. The unique characteristics of children with ASD can make their interactions with the immediate family and day-to-day household functioning just as challenging as their school, social events, and other types of interchange with the outside world.

In this chapter we offer a set of parenting strategies for handling common challenging behaviors that occur in the home, from resistance to homework and chores, to protests against changes in routine, to difficulty accepting household rules. We'll provide disciplinary strategies that acknowledge that children with ASD are motivated differently from other kids and often learn appropriate behavior via alternate routes. Then we'll look at typically difficult times of the day, such as bedtime, and tell you how to establish routines that will ease transitions and help your child fit neatly into daily family life.

Of course, your child with high-functioning ASD is not the only member of your family who needs attention. Our work with parents has taught us that attending to the personal needs of everyone in the family—parents and siblings included—is essential to maintaining a healthy family attitude and providing the most supportive environment for your child with ASD. So the second part of this chapter offers ideas for attending to your other children's needs—and your own—while handling the demanding task of caring for a child with the unique characteristics of ASD.

The Foundation: Consistency

As you've read throughout this book, and no doubt experienced in your own home, most children with ASD have a difficult time when their world is not consistent, routine, and predictable. As parents, therefore, you should always make consistency a priority, in both your overall approach to parenting and through the establishment of family routines and schedules. Making things consistent, routine, and predictable at home will reduce your child's confusion and anxiety and help promote positive behavior. In turn, this will help turn your home into a welcoming haven for the whole family. As we discussed in Chapter 5, many children with ASD have very strong memory and rule-following capabilities, which usually make them quite good at remembering and applying routines. This is a perfect opportunity to take advantage of your child's strengths on the home front.

Your efforts to maintain consistency in the home will be even more effective if your home rules and routines are the same as (or similar to) those established in other settings, such as the classroom. Taking on the task of working with teachers, baby-sitters, coaches, scout leaders, and other adults who may care for your child to make sure that all agree on a common set of rules and routines for your child to follow may seem daunting. But remember that, for a child with ASD, figuring out the rules is an arduous challenge, so this "one fell swoop" approach can be invaluable. Even if it proves impractical to have everyone echo exactly the same rules of behavior, you can ensure that certain dictates serve as consistent principles, such as "no hitting" and "no leaving the room [or the building] without adult permission." Children who learn that any physical aggression, for example, will be followed by a swift response from the adult in charge will begin to understand some basic principles of behavior that apply to all settings. This, in turn, frees up energy for figuring out the social nuances and skills that can be so difficult for kids with ASD to grasp on their own. You'll have to continue to help over time, communicating and working with teachers and service providers on a regular basis to remind everyone of the hierarchy of rules and of the framework for all routines.

Understanding Challenging Behavior

Some children with ASD occasionally display challenging behaviors, such as hitting, screaming, throwing tantrums, repetitive arguing, or even self-injury (such as slapping their own face or biting their hand). For many parents, particularly when you are in the midst of a "spirited episode" with your child, these problem behaviors seem like an end in and of themselves. You may get caught up in the moment, focusing on the idea that your child's objective is to engage in the challenging behavior and your goal is to squelch it. Obviously, you do need to deal with the immediate problem. However, it is important to remember that challenging behavior is not just random and almost always has a function or purpose. Most often, the child is trying to communicate his needs and wishes to others. So, if you want to discourage the challenging behavior, you need to determine what your child is trying to convey through it. Once you understand what he is trying to tell you, you can provide alternatives for expressing that want or need that are healthier and more appropriate for the setting. This is the foundation of an approach to behavior management called "functional behavior analysis," first introduced in Chapter 4, which is a systematic way of analyzing the purposes of difficult behavior so as to devise strategies for reducing them. Here are the steps involved in functional behavior analysis, with suggestions for using them to help your child eliminate challenging behavior. Incidentally, these steps should be used whenever problem behaviors erupt, whether in the home, at school, in the workplace, or in the neighborhood. For the sake of consistency, the following steps should be used not only by parents but also by teachers, therapists, and others who encounter the problem behavior in other settings.

Step 1: Try to Figure Out What Your Child Is Communicating with the Challenging Behavior

Common things that children try to tell us through their difficult behaviors include the following:

- Messages indicating that the child is confused and needs assistance:
    "This is too difficult for me."
    "This is confusing for me."
    "I can't remember what I am supposed to do."
- Messages expressing a feeling:
    "I'm hungry."
    "I'm sick."
    "I'm mad/sad/scared."
- Messages indicating that the child wants to escape from the current situation:
    "I don't like this and want to quit."
    "This situation is too stimulating for me."
    "I need some personal space."
    "When will I be done? How long will this go on?"

- Messages indicating that the child has a strong need for sameness, predictability, and routine:

    "I feel overwhelmed by these new [or unstructured] activities."

    "I expected things to be the same as before."

    "I don't want to stop doing what I am doing [for example, favorite activity]."

    "I'm not sure what happens next."

- Messages indicating that the child wants to access something or socially engage with someone but doesn't know how:

    "Give me that [object, item, food]."

    "I'm bored and want your attention."

    "I want to play with you."

When your child behaves inappropriately, ask yourself if you can hear any of these messages in the behavior. As parents, you know your child better than anyone else and have perhaps experienced her problem behaviors across many different settings for many years. Instinctively, you may have a very good idea of what your child is trying to communicate. But it's not always that easy. Here are some suggestions to make the process of understanding the behavior's function easier. These suggestions are based on the actual process used by professionals trained in functional behavior analysis.

Pay attention to the circumstances and contexts in which these difficult behaviors occur. Note also the consequences that result from the behavior. Write these down over the course of a week and then look for consistencies and themes. It may be helpful to use a piece of paper divided into three columns to record your observations. In the left-hand column, describe the situation or context that immediately preceded the occurrence of the behavior. In the middle column, describe the behavior. In the right-hand column, record what followed the behavior.

Here is an example:

Situation	Behavior	Consequence
Oct. 9, 7:30 P.M. I told Michael to turn off the TV and get ready for bed	Michael began crying and hitting the couch	I turned off the TV and dragged him kicking and fussing into his bedroom
Oct. 10, 6:30 P.M., dinnertime	Michael was making silly noises and faces	I asked him to leave the table
Oct. 10, 8:10 P.M., TV room, told Michael it was time for bed	Michael hit himself in the head and shouted "I hate going to bed"	I brought out his pajamas and prompted him to get dressed
Oct. 11, after school, Michael's sister had a friend over	Michael hit his sister and shoved her friend	His sister called me and I put him in time-out
Oct. 12, 6:00 P.M., sitting around the dinner table	Michael pinched his sister	His sister yelled "Stop it," Michael smiled, Dad asked Michael how far he got in his video game that day

After you've done this for several days, some clear themes may emerge. Are certain times of day or certain contexts often listed on the chart? Are the challenging behaviors that arise similar or different? You may notice that the behaviors themselves differ from day to day but the situations in which they arise are similar. Michael often has trouble at dinner, but also when his sister has a friend over. Are there any commonalities across those situations? Look at the list of five possibilities above and take some educated guesses about which is most plausible. Perhaps Michael needs more attention in these situations, or maybe he wants to interact but doesn't quite know how to. Michael also is easily upset when it is time to get ready for bed. Maybe he needs more help or doesn't want to make the transition away from his favorite pastime of watching TV. These hypotheses provide some good clues for how to change the behavior, which we will come to next.

If your child is mature enough, another method of making your guess is to check in with your child. Many children with ASD will have a hard time articulating complex feelings on their own, but they may be willing and able to communicate their motivations if you facilitate it by providing them with a list or multiple-choice questions. For example, when asked why she refused to speak to one of her care providers, one adolescent with high-functioning ASD wouldn't give any clear responses. But when provided with a list of items (with some comical ones thrown in for good measure) and asked to rank the reasons she was giving the person the cold shoulder, she was able to make her motivations clear. This strategy enabled her therapist to understand the motivations for her behaviors and to collaborate in forming a plan to make interactions with the care provider more appealing.

Step 2: Consider How You Can Change the Situation So That Your Child Will Be Less Likely to Need to Express His or Her Message in the First Place

Here are some examples of how a situation might be changed so that the need to communicate the messages listed above is reduced or eliminated altogether.

• If your child is expressing confusion or difficulty comprehending a situation, consider how you can make the situation easier to understand and more concrete, routine, or predictable. For example, you may need to simplify the task (break it into small steps or reduce the scope of expectations), repeat and simplify instructions, or offer visual supports such as written instructions or pictures to communicate what is expected.

- If your child is expressing a feeling or an unpleasant physiological state, try to remedy the situation. Feed him, take his temperature, get an appointment with your doctor to check for a disagreeable side effect from medication, or make sure he gets plenty of sleep.

- If your child is expressing that she is overwhelmed, overstimulated, and/or wants to escape a situation, consider avoiding this type of situation or reducing the amount of time spent in it whenever possible. If the situation is unavoidable, try to alter the most aversive aspects of the activity so that your child will find it more acceptable. Provide ample warning ahead of time and let your child know, using words or pictures, that a positive reward and/or break will be provided after the difficult situation ends.

Every Sunday morning, Amalia's complaining and repetitive talk began to crescendo as her family got into the car to head to church. Her parents knew that the length of the service and the crowd in the church were stressful for her. She had difficulty articulating her feelings on the subject, so she tended to act out to try to delay attending church. She also frequently asked to go to the bathroom during the service. Her parents made a rule that if she could make it through the service with two or fewer interruptions, they would stop by her favorite ice cream parlor on the way home. They even clipped out a picture of her favorite sundae so she could hold on to it during church to remind herself of her goal. After keeping a chart like the one described in Step 1 for two Sundays in a row, they also realized that Amalia's bathroom requests came just as the choir started singing. So the family began to sit in the back of the church, as far from the choir as possible, and allowed Amalia to wear earplugs when the singing began.

- If your child is having problems transitioning from one activity (typically a preferred activity) to another, make sure there are cues to indicate the upcoming transition (such as a picture or written schedule showing the order of activities). Provide plenty of advance warning (for example, by using a timer) and allow your child to have closure on the current activity (for example, by putting things away in a box, completing a computer game, and so on). Clarify what happens next and assist your child with making the transition by walking him through it.

> After filling in the chart in Step 1 for a week, Michael's mother noticed that getting ready for bed was a particularly difficult time. She would ask him to stop watching TV and get ready for bed, even giving him a warning to allow him time to finish his favorite TV program. But, inevitably, he would then become very distressed, start engaging in repetitive talk, such as asking questions about the previous TV show, cry, and sometimes even become aggressive. He would calm down only if she stopped what she was doing and walked him through each of the steps needed to get ready for bed. It occurred to her that perhaps the frustration and distress he had shown earlier were his way of communicating that he needed help with his bedtime routine. She realized that, although each step of the routine, such as brushing his teeth and putting on his pajamas, in itself was not difficult for Michael, sequencing the steps and completing them independently was quite challenging for him. Because Michael was a proficient reader, she decided to make a chart outlining the series of steps required for the bedtime routine and to encourage him to check off each step as he completed it. This not only helped him sequence and organize his behavior, but also gave him a sense of accomplishment.

• If your child's challenging behavior may indicate a desire for attention or to engage socially with another child, be sure to provide ample opportunities for social activities, such as organized clubs. Notice whether other children are responding positively to your child's attempts to initiate interaction when they are appropriate. If your child is being ignored, consider ways in which you can facilitate more positive responses to your child (such as structuring a one-on-one play date, as described in Chapter 8). If your child is trying to obtain a desired object, provide access to it whenever possible or devise a plan whereby your child could earn access by completing other less favored activities first.

Rashan loved to play on the computer, but he tended to ask to use it many times a day. If his parents didn't immediately respond by providing access to the computer, he would ask repetitively, sometimes hundreds of times in an hour, "When can I use it?" His parents truly thought they would be driven crazy! Following the "nothing of value should be given freely" adage (see Chapter 5), they decided to allow Rashan to use the computer 10 times a day, but always following a less preferred activity, such as doing 10 minutes of homework, loading the dishwasher, or brushing his teeth. Rashan was pleased to use the computer so often, and his demanding litany dropped in frequency.

Step 3: If the Message Must Be Communicated, Come Up with a Way in Which Your Child Can Communicate His or Her Needs or Wishes by Using a More Appropriate Behavior

If you can't eliminate the need for the message (as in Step 2), you need to help your child come up with more positive and acceptable ways of telling you what she needs to tell you. These include both appropriate verbal statements and more positive nonverbal ways to communicate the message and supplant the inappropriate behavior:

• Instead of screaming when confused by his homework, your child can be taught to raise his hand, ring a bell, turn sideways in his seat, or engage in some other nonverbal behavior that signals he needs help.

- Instead of biting her hand when asked to set the table, your child can learn to say, "I need help with this" or "This is too hard."

- Instead of hitting other people when he is distressed and wants to escape a situation, your son can say, "I don't like this."

- Instead of crying and hitting furniture when asked to turn off the TV and get ready for bed, your child can say, "I want to finish this show before I put on my pajamas."

- Instead of touching another child as a way of initiating interaction, your child can learn to say, "May I play too?"

- Instead of cursing and tearing up materials, your child can be taught to hold up a picture of a stop sign when he needs a break.

Whenever Eduardo became frustrated or bored during his homework, he would simply get up and leave the room and then resist coming back. His mother felt that he needed some breaks during homework time but was worried that taking too much time off would mean he'd never finish his assignments. She gave him five index cards, each of which said, "Good for One 3-Minute Break," and told him that from now on all he had to do was say, "I need a break," and he would immediately get a 3-minute respite. Just knowing this "out" was available to him made Eduardo feel that his homework was more manageable. Although it took a great deal of practice and prompting for Eduardo to learn to request a break on his own, this strategy was eventually very successful in helping him meet his needs in an appropriate way. As time wore on, Eduardo's mother was able to reduce the number of break cards from five to two. She also progressively lengthened the time between when Eduardo requested the break and when he actually took it, saying "OK, you can have a break after two [or three or six] more problems." In this way, she balanced the need to honor Eduardo's new, more appropriate communication with the necessity that he still get his homework done.

Step 4: Practice the New Way of Communicating

How to practice:

- Model for your child the more appropriate phrase or non-verbal signal she can use to communicate needs or desires.

- Have your child practice the new phrase or behavior before the situation in which it is likely to be needed takes place.

- During the situation, remind (prompt) your child to use the new phrase or behavior.

> Vincent had a habit of shoving peers when they approached a toy he was playing with on the playground. His mother taught him to say, "I'm playing with this now. You can have it when I'm done." To help Vincent learn how to use this skill, she modeled the behavior, having Vincent approach her and try to touch a toy she was using. Next, she helped him do the same as she approached his toy. Then she accompanied him to the playground and observed him as he played near other children. When she saw a situation arising in which Vincent was likely to hit a peer, she reminded him to say the phrase they had practiced. When Vincent used the phrase, she made sure that the peer responded positively by ceasing his request for the toy. Finally, she talked to Vincent's teacher about using the same procedure in the classroom and at recess, so that they would all be addressing his inappropriate behavior consistently. The teacher agreed to practice using the phrase with Vincent at school and follow up by prompting him whenever necessary.

Step 5: Reward Your Child for Using the Strategy by Showing That It Gets His or Her Needs Met

You must make sure the new communication strategy you've taught your child is as effective as the old one. If screaming or repetitive complaining is more effective than saying "I want to finish this video" or holding up a break card, your child will have little moti-vation to use the new strategy. Whenever possible, immediately reward your child for using the appropriate communication, first by praising him ("I'm glad you're using your new words") and then by "honoring the communication" and making sure the natural positive consequences occur:

- When your child requests help, immediately assist her.
- If your child asks to leave a situation, provide him with a break right away.
- If your child asks for your attention, stop what you're doing and provide some time, interest in, and engagement with her.

Your child will learn that these new, appropriate behaviors are just as effective or even more effective in meeting his needs than the challenging behaviors you are trying to reduce.

Step 6: Be Sure That the Challenging Behavior Is No Longer Effective in Getting Your Child's Needs Met

Leave your child no alternative for getting her needs met besides the new, appropriate method you've taught. Ignore the problem behavior whenever it occurs, but provide a prompt for the new communication. For example, if your child screams whenever she wants to avoid a situation, prompt her to use an appropriate phrase, but do not permit her to leave the situation while she is screaming.

Ivana's 11-year-old daughter, Michaela, had a habit of coming up to her siblings and classmates and touching them to get their attention. When she was younger, this type of behavior seemed appropriate, even affectionate. But now that she was approaching adolescence her mother was concerned that it would irritate peers and could lead to erroneous signals being sent to boys. Ivana explained to Michaela why this behav-ior was not appropriate and taught her instead to say, "Hi, how's it going?" Ivana modeled and role-played this skill with Michaela, and she also talked to her other children about the strategy. She asked them to ignore Michaela if she touched them but to pay attention to her right away if she asked for their attention as she had been taught. This ensured simultaneously that Michaela's inappropriate skills would not be successful and that her new strategies would be rewarding.

The steps we've described are straightforward, but it is no easy task to switch your child from challenging behaviors to more appropriate means of attaining their desired goals. It will be crucial for you to practice with your child and to ensure that appropriate strategies will be more reinforcing than those based on difficult or inappropriate behaviors. Some parents have lamented that when they try to alter these challenging behaviors, they seem to increase in frequency. Although it may seem counterintuitive, this is actually a good sign. When children find that their old, tried-and-true strategy isn't working, they often take a "twice as much, twice as hard" approach in a last-ditch effort to achieve their goals. This indicates that your child has realized that the contingencies have changed. As long as you don't yield to this increased frequency and intensity of the problem behavior, change is probably imminent.

Strategies for Positive Discipline

As you may have experienced with your own child, many standard disciplinary methods don't work well with children who have ASD. They often do not have good self-monitoring skills and may lack the ability to judge whether their behavior is appropriate. They may not pick up on cues that normally would signal that their behavior does not fit in, and they may not feel the embarrassment or shame that many children experience when they have behaved inappropriately. Nor are they always motivated by a desire to please their parents and other adults by behaving well.

When 10-year-old Ronald had his friends over, they would try to talk with Ronald's 14-year-old brother, Peter, to ask him about a video game he had mastered. Peter had no interest in talking with his brother's friends, but because he had ASD, he didn't know how to communicate his feelings appropriately and would simply shove Ronald and his friends out of the way. Peter's mother would then send Peter to his room for shoving his brother's friends, which actually rewarded his inappropriate behavior by providing him with the solitude he wanted.

Approaches like time-out, which work well for a typically developing child, may fall short with your child with ASD. In general, the following strategies are more useful for children with ASD:

• Establish a set of concrete rules and be consistent in enforcing them.

• Make sure your child knows what is expected of him by writing it down or even illustrating it with pictures. Tasks such as dressing, brushing teeth, and setting the table may need to be broken down into small steps. It may be helpful to visually describe these steps in either pictorial or written form. If your child responds best to pictures, use a camera to photograph each step needed to complete a task and post the photos in your child's room or another area of the house.

• Describe your expectations in terms of what your child is supposed to do, rather than what she is not supposed to do: "Keep your hands in your lap," rather than "Do not hit." This makes your commands more positive and prevents a pattern of nagging from forming. More practically, it cements in your child's mind a constructive alternative behavior for future use.

• Establish a morning and an evening routine. If necessary, outline the routine in words or pictures (often called an "activity schedule"—see the example in Chapter 4). Set clear boundaries for activities and signal their beginning and end by using timers or visual cues (for example, by putting play materials away in a container). Provide concrete cues that an activity is coming to an end (for example, by saying "The timer is about to ring and then you need to turn off the computer").

• Use preferred activities as rewards for completing nonpreferred activities (for example, "Once you have brushed your teeth, you can read your dinosaur book").

• Limit the time your child engages in nonproductive preoccupations by setting explicit rules. For example, your child may ask you three questions per evening about his favorite topic or may play on the computer for a specific amount of time each evening.

Strategies for Difficult Times of the Day

Mornings

Mornings are a particularly difficult time for most families. During this period of transition from sleeping to waking and from home to school, children are particularly vulnerable to problems with over- and underarousal. For many children who find school a stressful experience, the morning is also a time of anticipatory distress and last-ditch escape maneuvers. A helpful strategy is to accomplish as much preparation as possible the night before so that morning moods are less likely to interfere with the routine. For example, by laying clothes out prior to bedtime and organizing school materials by the front door, you can eliminate two tasks from the morning routine.

It may be useful to experiment with different approaches to waking your child to ease the transition from sleep to alertness. See if your child reacts differently to being awakened by a person, a buzzer, or a radio. Some parents find it helpful to give "incremental" alarms, alerting their child that she will have to get up in 10 minutes and then warning her again 5 minutes before actually asking the child to get out of bed.

Mealtimes

Meals are also often a hard time for families of children with ASD. Many such children are finicky eaters, and this problem can be compounded by special diets or sensitivities to certain consistencies and textures. Many parents begin to worry about a picky child's nutritional intake, and, as they make this a focus of attention, the child perceives this as an opportunity for control. In this circumstance, mealtimes can turn into a real power struggle. Many parents find it helpful to introduce new foods one food at a time and one bite at a time. For some children, an even slower pace might be appropriate. For example, you might proceed from tolerating new foods on the table or plate to smelling the food, touching the food with the fingers, touching the food to the lips, licking the food, placing it in the mouth, and finally chewing and swallowing it. Many children will not accept a new food until it has been introduced several times. Some research studies suggest that changes in eating habits may take 2 weeks or longer to be observable. So be patient and allow your child adequate time to adjust to something new.

If you are seriously concerned that your child's nutritional intake may be insufficient, there are several steps you can take. First, check your child's height and weight with your pediatrician. Is your child's growth in the reasonably appropriate range? If there is cause for concern, keep a log of what your child eats (be sure to get information about what he eats at school) and seek consultation with a nutritionist. It is particularly important to receive nutritional consultation before implementing a special diet.

It is also essential to keep in mind that parents don't always get an accurate impression of what their child eats. The mother of Sandra, an 8-year-old girl with high-functioning ASD, was under the impression that her daughter ate nothing but pretzels and cheese. After consulting with the doctor and finding out that her height and weight parameters were appropriate, she asked Sandra's teacher about her eating habits at school. She learned that Sandra regularly ate the entire school lunch, including vegetables and milk.

It is also helpful to keep meals consistent in terms of time of day. This helps your child know what to expect and allows meals to be incorporated into a regular routine. For some children, it may even be helpful to create a meal schedule or weekly menu to make meals predictable. When it is time for a meal, serve your child's food with the rest of the family's food (assuming your family has the luxury of dining together each evening). If your child chooses not to eat when the rest of the family is at the table, make it clear that she may lose the opportunity to eat dinner that evening. This practice forces your child to adhere to a meal schedule, which helps a sometimes dysregulated body ease into a healthy eating pattern. It also capitalizes on your child's desire for rules. If a clear rule is set (for example, "Everyone eats together"), then it is more likely that your child will embrace it.

For children who tend to get up from the table, seating them against a wall can be helpful. This makes it slightly more difficult for them to wander and increases the chance that they will stay put. You can also use strategies such as those described above in the section "Understanding Challenging Behavior." What function does the wandering seem to serve? Would providing a few short breaks during dinner help? Would a timer that shows how much longer your child needs to sit help? Would it help to provide your child with conversation topics or scripts (see Chapter 8) for the dinner table, so that he would be able to interact more appropriately with family members? Would it help to provide your child with something to hold in his hand or squeeze under the table while he waits for the others to finish?

After-School Time

The period after school is another difficult transition time for many children with ASD. There is no absolute rule regarding the most appropriate after-school activity; however, the principle of consistency applies here as well. As a parent, you are the expert on your child. Is school a taxing experience for your child, and does she require some "alone time" to decompress after the stressful day? Or does your energetic child need some time to run around and expend energy after being forced to sit in one place for so many hours? Is your child in an academic rhythm by the end of the school day, and should you "go with the flow" and do homework upon arrival at home? Think of what the most appropriate after-school activity is for your child and keep it consistent from day to day.

Bedtime

Another challenging transition, bedtime, can be a daunting endeavor, especially since studies have shown that ASD is often associated with sleep difficulties. Bedtime routines, such as going to bed at the same time and engaging in the same prebedtime tasks, are helpful for all children, but especially for those with ASD. Give your child plenty of advance warning and a countdown (30 minutes, 20 minutes, and so on) as bedtime approaches. To help your child wind down, make sure he engages in a quiet activity, like reading or playing a mellow game, before bedtime. Another strategy for ensuring "decompression" time is to spend some time with your child in his bedroom before you turn out the lights and expect him to go to sleep. If you sit with your child at bedtime, make sure you are consistent in the amount of time you spend at the bedside. Be sure that your presence is not serving as stimulation that keeps your child awake. Some children find it reassuring to know that after they have fallen asleep, you will check on them.

Make sure the bedroom is a pleasant place for your child. For some children, it is important to keep favorite belongings in the room. For others, it can be excessively distracting or overstimulating. Some children find the presence of soft light or music sooth-ing, while others require complete darkness and absolute silence to fall asleep.

If you try these suggestions and still find that your child has sleep difficulties, you should consider checking with your pediatri-cian, who may suggest other techniques or medications to help your child with sleep. Chapter 4 contains some additional tips for creating behavioral and visual routines for bedtime.

Family Outings

For most family members, outings and vacations are fun and excit-ing. For the child with ASD, however, family outings may mean a break in routine, unpredictability, unfamiliarity, and the need to deal with new people and places. For these reasons, they can be anxiety-provoking times for children with ASD. Parents can mini-mize stress by planning in advance and letting the child know what it will be like. Try Carol Gray's Social Story approach, which involves showing your child a story consisting of pictures depicting the experience and words describing what will happen. (Chapter 8 describes how to use this approach in detail.) For a child who is apprehensive about a planned family outing to an amusement park, you might visit the amusement park's website and print out some images of the parking lot, the entrance gate, and some of the rides. Then you can write a simple story to accompany the pic-tures that helps your child know what to anticipate. Read the story together several times before your family actually ventures out to the park. There are many preprinted Social Stories available that are appropriate for both recreational and nonrecreational activi-ties, such as visits to the doctor. The Resources at the end of the book contain information about Social Stories.

It may be necessary to acclimate your child to a new experience slowly by gradually introducing it in small steps. After reviewing the new experience using visual cues such as a Social Story ahead of time, you may want to arrange a short visit to the new place or activity. Over time, your child is likely to feel more comfortable with the new activity, at which point you can lengthen your visit.

Chores and Household Responsibilities

Encouraging children to help around the home is a challenge for every parent, including those parenting children with high-functioning ASD. It is typical for children to dislike chores and to try their best to shirk these responsibilities in lieu of something more fun. To make chores more tolerable for a child with ASD, embed them in a daily or weekly routine. This consistency will help your child know what needs to be done and prevent a chore from being an unwelcome surprise. Likewise, try to routinize the steps in the chore. Capitalizing on their typical visual strengths, many children will be helped by creating a written checklist or set of pictures that outlines the steps involved in the task. For example, to help a child with taking out the garbage, show pictures of a person removing the garbage bag, tying it, placing it in the can in the garage, and then putting in a new bag. Work through the list with your child several times to help her learn the steps involved.

Choosing appropriate tasks is a crucial factor in assigning chores, as we discussed in the last chapter. When first introducing the idea of household responsibilities to your child, start out with a task that is simple and easy to accomplish. Whenever possible, choose tasks that are naturally suited to your child's strengths.

Evan is a 12-year-old boy with ASD and a preference for order in his physical environment. He has four typically developing siblings, and his home often looks as though a tornado has just passed through. His mother decided to assign him the task of organizing the furniture and coffee table in the living room once a day. Evan initially resisted taking on this responsibility, but he reluctantly agreed when he realized it could earn him additional computer time. It soon became clear to his mother that restoring order to the living room actually had a calming effect on Evan. The arrangement enabled him to help out around the house, soothe himself, and earn privileges.

For older children, parents may wish to assign chores that provide practice for skills applicable in a job, such as filing, washing dishes, and preparing the ingredients for cooking.

Homework

Make a structured homework schedule so that your child completes homework at the same time and in the same place every day. Actually putting this information on a visual schedule is helpful. It reminds the child about what is coming and also helps the child remember that something more fun will happen after homework is complete. For some children, it may be necessary to further structure the homework session. When a child receives a number of different assignments, he may find it challenging to determine the best way to approach the tasks. If your child finds the prospect confusing, help out by making a list of what needs to be done with what priorities. By laying out a concrete plan of attack, you can make the task seem much less overwhelming to children. Chapter 7 contains more detailed suggestions for organizing academic tasks, including homework, for your child.

Many children with ASD are easily distracted. Therefore, they need a workplace that is free from distractions, including noise, clutter, and other family members. Tailor an approach that is appropriate to the attentional capacities and working style of your child. For some children, it is best to complete all homework in a single sitting. Other children find this excessively taxing and may benefit from breaks in between smaller work periods. One parent we worked with sets a kitchen timer for her child. For 30 minutes of productive homework, the child earns a 5-minute computer break. Or you might give your child a break after each assignment or subject is finished. Providing a break or other type of positive reinforcement (maybe a special food treat or a token that can be redeemed for bigger rewards), during or upon completion of homework, will increase your child's motivation. Parents can also make use of the reinforcing properties of homework itself. Many children with ASD are extremely enthusiastic about particular school subjects. Completing favorite homework last serves as reinforcement for working on less interesting subject matter earlier.

Be conscious of the influence that your child's motor and sensory characteristics may have on the homework process. For many children with ASD, handwriting is a difficult fine motor task. The physical difficulty of writing out homework can make the task even more unpleasant. Try to be as creative and flexible as possible in solving these types of problems. For example, ask your child's teacher if she could complete the assignment on a computer or dictate the answers rather than write them out (more on these topics in Chapter 7). Children's sensory sensitivities also influence the completion of homework. For some individuals with ASD, reading under certain lighting conditions can be difficult. Experiment with light levels and see what is most comfortable for your child.

Since homework bridges the gap between home and school, the idea of consistency between settings is particularly important. By communicating with your child's teacher, you can learn about strategies that have been successful at school and share techniques that have worked in the home. Communication between parents and teachers also fosters consistency in terms of the rules associated with homework completion. If your child's teacher permits breaks every 20 minutes, you should use the same schedule at home, rather than a 30-minute break interval. If the teacher reinforces correct work with stickers or check marks, rather than tokens, use those instead. As we mentioned earlier in this chapter, when a child has a single set of rules to follow across multiple settings, he has a much easier time knowing what is expected and is more likely to behave accordingly.

Having someone else assist your child with homework, perhaps an academic tutor you hire or a teacher in school, can be very helpful. Some children with ASD work so slowly that they bring home a great deal of homework. You may find it helpful to request an extra study hall or extra time in the resource room to help your child get more homework done at school. A designated person to help your child structure an approach to homework and to help with the actual completion of homework assignments can be a valuable support. This eliminates one potential area of difficulty that parents must negotiate with their child and also provides parents with some "down time" of their own after a long workday, be it in an office or in the home. Many tutors with experience in working with children with ASD are available, and they can help devise novel strategies for working with your child. Your local autism society probably maintains a list of tutors. Or check with the pediatrics or child psychiatry department of your local hospital or the agency at which your child was diagnosed.

Maintaining a Healthy Family Attitude

Siblings

Working to ensure the psychological well-being of the siblings of children with ASD is one of the most valuable investments parents can make. With a healthy attitude, siblings can be a parent's greatest allies in caring for a child with ASD. They can also be great friends to and serve as role models for children with ASD, particularly for helping them understand the social world. Finally, of course, when they are happy and feel supported, siblings contribute to the overall well-being of the whole family.

For some typically developing children who have siblings with special needs, there doesn't seem to be much cause for concern. Claire, the older sister of a boy with ASD, stated, "Just because Clark has special needs doesn't mean that I do too." Her unwavering love for her brother and her candor with peers rendered it an insignificant issue for her. She felt so comfortable around people with ASD that she sought out other opportunities, such as volunteering at the Special Olympics, and sometimes even brought her friends along with her. They all felt enriched by the experiences, and both Claire and one of her friends eventually went into careers that involved helping children with special needs.

Unfortunately, however, for many children a sibling with ASD presents a host of familial, social, and personal challenges.

Communicating with Siblings

The most important principles in dealing with siblings of children with ASD are honesty, education, and open-mindedness. Your typically developing child will likely have myriad questions about her sibling: Why doesn't he talk to me? Why does she do those weird things? How come he won't play with me? Does she hate me? Can I "catch" ASD? Does my brother have ASD because I wrestled too hard with him when he was a baby? The more your typically developing child understands about ASD, the greater the insight into her sibling and the less likely that misconceptions, such as those regarding contagion or causality, can contribute to stress. Make sure to create time for open, honest, nonjudgmental discussions when your child can discuss feelings, both positive and negative, regarding her sibling with ASD. In these conversations, probe your child regarding her experiences at home and at school. What are the issues she doesn't understand? What positive and negative aspects of having a brother or sister with ASD has she experienced recently? As a parent, you can set an excellent example, being positive and accepting of your child's special needs, but also making clear that sometimes frustration or other negative emotion is unavoidable. A recent study showed that even after parents had talked with their typically developing children about ASD, most of the siblings harbored many misconceptions or didn't understand some basics of the condition. In other words, just because you explain something to your typically developing child, it doesn't mean that she has comprehended what you have said. Asking your typically developing child to explain in her own words what you have said may be helpful. And having frequent, ongoing discussions, rather than only a few brief conversations, is needed.

A positive approach to facilitating communication with your typically developing child is to include him in discussions of how best to help your child with ASD. This is not appropriate for children at all developmental levels, but mature children and adolescents can contribute excellent insights to the experiences of their sibling with ASD and the causes of certain behaviors. As a peer, the sibling may also have helpful opinions about social relationship strategies and school settings. By including your typically developing child in the process, you foster family unity and prevent anyone from feeling excluded.

Guilt and Excessive Responsibility

Some siblings of children with special needs can be excessively demanding of themselves. They might try to help out to the extent that their own schoolwork or social life suffers. Some psychologists speak of the "little parent" effect, in which a typical sibling starts behaving more like a caregiving adult than a child. You can help prevent this from occurring by being careful not to rely too much on your typical child's assistance in caring for the sibling with ASD at home or at school.

Typical siblings can also become emotionally vulnerable because of their own thought processes. A certain degree of tension between siblings is natural, even adaptive, in that it provides a forum for learning to resolve conflicts with others. However, a well-intentioned sibling of a child with special needs may experience guilt regarding negative feelings toward a sibling who "just can't help it." Try to help your child understand that these feelings are natural and that what is most important is how he acts on them. It is OK, even normal, to resent a brother or sister who requires much of Mom and Dad's attention or who seems to have much lower demands made on him or her. Let your typically developing children know that you understand these thoughts, perhaps even share them sometimes, and that you love them just the same as if all their thoughts of their sibling were warm and positive. Be clear that it is OK to have these thoughts as long as they are not acted on in a harmful or negative way.

Equal Attention, Activity, and Discipline

A common perception of typically developing siblings is that brothers and sisters with ASD receive disproportionate amounts of parental attention. Very often, this may be the case. There is no getting around the fact that children with ASD have special needs and may require additional attention to accomplish things typically developing children can do easily. Nevertheless, there are several strategies you can use to prevent siblings' feelings of neglect and potential resentment. In two-parent homes, divide and conquer, splitting up so that you can attend to two children simultaneously. In one-parent families, calling on the assistance of friends or relatives to help out can provide additional caregivers and allow you more flexibility in distributing your time. It is important to be honest and straightforward and to acknowledge your devotion to your typically developing child and your commitment to making sure that all the wheels, not just the squeaky ones, get some grease. Take some time each day to devote your full attention to your typically developing children, even if only briefly. During bedtime routines or other evening activities, make sure that you ask your typically developing children about their experiences, feelings, and concerns. Designate a day once or twice a month that will be devoted to your typical child's interests and find someone else to take care of your child with ASD on those days. This type of gesture goes a long way in making clear that all your children are important to you.

This last strategy relates to another common sentiment among siblings of children with ASD, the notion that the child's special needs will restrict the activities of the entire family. Take the example of a family outing to a combination pizzeria/arcade. For many children this is about as fun as it gets, but for some children with ASD the noise, visual stimulation, and crowds of people can be overwhelming. It is easy for a parent to avoid such activities to suit the needs of the family member with ASD. However, this practice can foster resentment in typical children. It also reduces the range of experiences encountered by your child with ASD and may reinforce her behavioral inflexibility. For this reason, it is essential that you plan a variety of activities that encompass everyone's interests. Allowing the preferences of your child with ASD to dictate family experiences is a dangerous but easy routine to fall into.

Discipline is another area in which it can be difficult to be fair to all of your children. It is sometimes necessary to have different rules and expectations for your child with ASD. This can quite easily foster the impression in typical siblings that a brother or sister with special needs is allowed to misbehave with seeming impunity. There are two strategies for confronting this problem. The first is to critically evaluate your application of disciplinary rules. Maybe your child is right and you are making it a bit easier on your child with ASD. Examine house rules to make sure any discrepancies in expectation across siblings are genuinely necessary. For example, if your typical child has to do chores to earn privileges, make sure your child with ASD has household responsibilities too, even if they are more basic. Second, when differences exist with justifiable reason, explain the situation to your typical child. A child who understands the reasons for disparities is less likely to resent parents and affected siblings.

Peer Relationships

Many parents express concern regarding the effects that a child with ASD might have on siblings' peer relationships. We've found that peers' responses can range from cruel to caring. Teaching your typical child to explain ASD to others and to express his feelings about the subject provides tools for interacting with others on this topic in more comfortable ways. Although it will be important to consult with your typical child before doing so, it can help to invite over some friends from school to meet the affected sibling. This serves to quench their curiosity and help them gain a more realistic perception of ASD. Once classmates understand what their friend's brother or sister is like, they are more likely to act as allies if others are behaving inappropriately and will be more accessible and informed sources of support for your typically developing child. They will also grow up to be more caring, compassionate adults who tolerate diversity.

Some parents find it necessary to set boundaries regarding interaction between an affected sibling and a typical sibling's friends. There's a delicate balance between giving the child with ASD the benefit of social exposure and allowing your typical child to feel independent in her friendships. Create certain times when all the children can interact together, for example, by serving a snack or by allowing them to play video games or sports in a group. Also ensure that your typical child has the opportunity to be alone with her friends. Some parents find it helpful to make a rule that when children are in common space it is common time, but when friends go into a child's room, it becomes personal time. Respecting your typical child's friendships is important to promote both healthy social development and maintenance of a positive attitude toward the family and affected siblings.

Personal Life

We've already discussed strategies for accommodating household routines to your child with ASD. The same policy is important for your typically developing child. Try to be aware of how your child with ASD affects the household experience of your other children. Is the affected child making too much noise when siblings are trying to sleep or do homework? Make sure you respect the habits and needs of all members of the family.

We've heard numerous children complain about their sibling with ASD taking their belongings and failing to respect their personal space. Given the difficulties children with ASD experience in judging personal boundaries and inferring the sentiments of others, it is important for you to intervene and make sure that your typical child has a "safe" space where prized possessions or personal items can be kept away from prying eyes and probing hands. This space can be a drawer, a closet, or even a room that is off limits to his sibling. In addition to the practical advantage of providing your child with a safe spot, it sends a clear message that you are keeping your typical child's interests in mind. When implementing this idea, be consistent and provide your ASD child with a special and safe space for his treasures too!

Additional Support

There are several books that focus specifically on sibling issues. *Siblings of Children with Autism: A Guide for Families*, by Sandra Harris and Beth Glasberg, provides specific strategies for teaching children about ASD and helping them communicate their experiences on the subject. A number of age-appropriate books and websites are designed to help siblings of children with ASD grapple with the unique challenges the situation presents (see Resources). Sometimes counseling is a helpful source of support for the typically developing child experiencing difficulty coming to terms with her sibling's disability. Support groups specifically designed for siblings of children with ASD exist in certain parts of the country (*www.siblingsupport.org/sibshops*). These groups provide a comfortable, friendly setting for children to learn from and make friends with others who have had similar experiences.

Parents as People

ASD is recognized as one of the most difficult diagnoses for parents to come to terms with. Perhaps because we know so little about its causes, many parents instinctively feel a sense of guilt. Depression in parents after receiving the diagnosis is not uncommon. Marital relationships are strained, resulting in higher than average rates of divorce among families of children with special needs. Thus, it is important that you consider not only the needs of your children but also your own needs. You are the primary support for your child with ASD, and the healthier you are, the better support you will be able to provide.

One ingredient in taking care of yourself is to invest some time, even if it is just a few minutes after everyone is asleep, in personal activities that you enjoy, every day. Preserve your individual identity beyond being the parent of a child with special needs. Take turns with your spouse taking a night off once a week to pursue personal recreation or socialize with friends. If you are a single parent, try to arrange for a babysitter or friend to care for your children once a week so you can take a break for personal socializing or other individual pursuits.

Just as an individual's mental health can suffer if it is neglected, a relationship requires similar attention. It can be very difficult for parents to preserve quality time with a partner. Continually neglecting the relationship can have adverse effects on everyone in the family, including the child you are working so hard to help. Many parents call on relatives or friends to watch the children for a few hours each week. Other parents hire respite providers to allow them a few hours of personal or social time. An essential means of minimizing stress in two-parent families is to thoroughly discuss and agree on treatment and parenting decisions, both to minimize discord and to achieve consistency. Sometimes this is difficult and you may find it necessary to involve a professional, such as your child's doctor or a therapist, to discuss different options and treatment decisions.

Maintaining adult relationships can be even more difficult when one of the partners is not the biological parent of the child with ASD. Single parents who are dating or in new relationships often feel torn about taking time away from their child. We can't stress enough that taking care of yourself rivals taking care of your child in importance. If you are lonely, unfulfilled, and in dire need of adult conversation, your patience and resources for your child with ASD will diminish. Try hard to carve out special time, away from your child, to interact with other adults, including romantic partners. You may find it helpful to provide information about ASD to new partners in small doses, if they appear interested. Encourage interactions with your child with ASD in structured circumstances that highlight his skills. The stereotypes of severe autism that many people hold, just because they know no better, are important to dispel for anyone who may become important in your life. Help others learn about the unique and interesting side of ASD. As you know, living with ASD is not always easy, but it is by no means always difficult either.

Whether yours is a one-parent or a two-parent family, you should take advantage of the numerous support groups that have been formed for parents of children with ASD. These groups can usually offer useful tips from parents who have encountered comparable challenges. Some groups also provide child care while parents meet, which gives parents some much needed "down time" and creates an informal social group for children with ASD. The most important benefit of support groups, however, is the opportunity to communicate with others who have survived the same struggles you are encountering. It can be very reassuring to realize your situation is not as extraordinary as it may often seem and to learn successful coping strategies from empathic peers.

If you can't find a support group in your area, consider creating an informal group yourself. Some parents who have met through their child's school or therapies have gone on to form informal support groups on their own. Meeting at a family's home once a month gives parents a chance to discuss issues and provide support for one another.

Managing a family with a child with ASD puts extra stress on everyone, to be sure. However, by using the strategies in this chapter, we hope your family can more easily focus on the opportunities for accomplishment, joy, and laughter that your special child can inspire as well.

7

High-Functioning Autism Spectrum Disorder at School

At age 8, Joseph is the best reader and speller in his third-grade class. He is also a whiz at computers and often is able to figure out the problem when his teacher has trouble logging on or opening folders. His teacher, who is very fond of Joseph and continually amazed at his talents, asks him to help a classmate who has had little experience with computers. Joseph beams as he demonstrates how to use the mouse and navigate the Internet. In a recent talent show, Joseph showed his class how he can read *The New York Times* upside down in a mirror. Joseph struggles in many other areas, however. He sometimes misinterprets what he reads and often can't answer simple questions about a paragraph that he has read aloud quickly and flawlessly. Joseph can subtract three-digit numbers in his head but can't figure out how much money he needs for lunch or whether he gets the right amount of change back. His handwriting is very poor, and he resists using a pencil, so his teacher allows him to use a keyboard for writing assignments. His desk is a horrible mess, with papers that he has forgotten to hand in, assignments he has never finished, old food, and little trinkets spilling out. He often appears as if he isn't listening or is absorbed in daydreams. When the teacher gives directions, Joseph sits quietly, lost in thought, while all around him his classmates get their workbooks out and turn to the page the teacher indicated. And Joseph often complains of boredom when the class studies topics that don't interest him (basically anything unrelated to geography). His parents have asked the teacher to modify some of his assignments so that they somehow involve geography, but the teacher is not sure whether this will go too far in "coddling" Joseph or making him stand out even further from his classmates.

When Hans Asperger first described children like Joseph, he highlighted both their special cognitive strengths and their serious academic weaknesses, saying that "these exceptional human beings must be given exceptional educational treatment. . . . These children raise questions of central importance to psychology and education." He and Leo Kanner, both of whom described what is now called ASD in the 1940s, recognized immediately that standard educational practices would not always work for children with ASD and that special measures would need to be taken to ensure that they achieved to their true potential. In this chapter, we outline a variety of different school services and accommodations that use the special strengths of the condition to help children and adolescents with high-functioning ASD succeed academically, despite the cognitive challenges that may also be present.

The Cognitive and Academic Profile
of Higher-Functioning Individuals with ASD

Chapter 5 reviewed the cognitive talents that are often part of ASD, and Chapter 2 introduced the cognitive challenges that are often part of the profile for ASD. Joseph exemplifies a typical (although not universal) pattern, in which some of his academic skills are highly advanced, others are age-appropriate, and still others are truly deficient. Joseph can sound out almost any word he is shown, but he doesn't always know what it means. This indicates a dissociation between his reading decoding and reading comprehension skills. Similarly, in math he understands the rules of addition and subtraction and is even beginning to memorize the multiplication tables, but he has trouble applying these skills to the real world and using them in a commonsense fashion. He often appears unmotivated to learn about things that other children are intrinsically interested in. Earning good grades and obtaining teacher and parent approval seem unimportant to Joseph.

One of Joseph's greatest sources of difficulty is his trouble with organization, planning, and goal-directed activities (often called "executive function" skills). Joseph frequently daydreams, which causes him to miss what the teacher is saying or what he is supposed to be doing. He is not distracted by external stimuli, however, as in the case of individuals with attention-deficit/ hyperactivity disorder (ADHD), but internally: he can get totally absorbed in his own thoughts and lose track of what is going on in the classroom. Joseph also has trouble managing time and works very slowly and methodically; consequently, he often falls behind during class, resulting in hours of homework in the evening. He can't seem to get organized: when he sits down to do homework, he has invariably forgotten something he needs to complete the assignment. Either he's left it at school or he goes off in search of it and gets distracted by something of higher interest and an hour elapses. Joseph's backpack is such a jumble that he can't find the homework he's done to turn it in—or else he just plain forgets that this last step is essential. In mid-February, he gave his family a Christmas ornament he had made in school as a holiday gift after discovering it at the bottom of his desk. Joseph tends to get bogged down in details and has trouble distinguishing what is most relevant from minor issues. He is prone to go off on tangents or to get overly focused on something unimportant. For example, when writing a book report, he spent so much time trying to figure out the author's date of birth that he wasn't able to complete the assignment, even though his mother stayed up until midnight to help him with it.

This profile of strengths and weaknesses is quite distinct from the learning disabilities that teachers are most often aware of. For example, children with dyslexia (reading disability), the most common learning disorder, demonstrate essentially the opposite pattern from Joseph. They are unable to sound out words due to a profound deficit in hearing speech sounds in language and difficulty learning how letters correspond to sounds. When asked to read aloud, they read haltingly and with great difficulty, mispronouncing, skipping, or guessing at many words. Despite these problems, children with dyslexia can often answer questions about what they've read perfectly—an uncanny ability considering all the reading errors they have made and the poor correspondence between the printed page and what they say aloud.

This is the kind of pattern that teachers learn about during their training and know how to address. But many teachers have never been faced with a student who can read a passage perfectly but has trouble understanding what it means. Likewise, organizational and planning difficulties are not typical forms of learning disability. Teachers often have trouble believing that a child who is bright in so many ways can "forget" about a long-planned field trip or fail to anticipate what materials are needed to complete an assignment. Because of the relative rarity of these academic difficulties, children with high-functioning ASD can frustrate even the most understanding teachers and parents. Occasionally this leads to misinterpretation of the child's behaviors and negative attributions about the student—for example, that he or she is lazy, stubborn, willfully disobedient, or defiant. Many teachers, and even some parents, have felt that the child "could do it if he [she] really wanted to." This can be a harmful attitude for the child. It not only can set up an adversarial relationship between the child and the teacher, but, even worse, may prevent the child from getting the services or accommodations he might need to succeed in school and later in life. Finally, this attitude can also have a negative effect on your child's self-esteem and feelings about school.

Learning Disabilities and ASD

The fact that there are major distinctions between the cognitive challenges posed by ASD and those posed by learning disabilities does not preclude the possibility that a child will have both. While it is relatively uncommon for children with ASD to have dyslexia too, it does occasionally happen. If your child is experiencing trouble with phonics (sounding out words), by all means have her evaluated for dyslexia. Most school psychologists and many clinical psychologists in the community are trained to perform these specialized evaluations.

A learning disability that occurs with more frequency among children with high-functioning ASD is known as nonverbal learning disability, or NLD. Children with NLD experience selective difficulty with mathematics, visual–spatial skills (for example, completing puzzles, mazes, drawing), and handwriting, but function fine when the activity relies primarily on language skills (for example, reading, spelling, answering questions). They are often clumsy and late to walk or to develop other motor skills, such as riding a bike. Many children with NLD have trouble reading the emotions of others and may have other social difficulties, such as shyness or trouble making friends. Some of these difficulties overlap with ASD (social problems and delayed motor skills, for example), while others are relatively rare in ASD (such as poor visual–spatial skills). To be diagnosed with NLD, a child must experience the hallmark cognitive and academic symptoms of the syndrome, including poor math and visual–spatial skills and lowered nonverbal intelligence; the social and motor symptoms alone are not enough for a diagnosis. If your child exhibits several of these difficulties, it is worth requesting an evaluation from your school to see if he would benefit from extra assistance in learning math or qualify for occupational therapy services.

Educational Services

Most children with ASD, even those who are high functioning, will need special educational services and accommodations at some point, if not throughout their schooling. One of the first questions raised by parents about educational services involves school placement. Would their child be better off in a regular or a special education classroom, in a public or a private school? The answers to these questions depend on the individual child: no placement or set of services is universally successful for all children with ASD. It is important for parents to know that special education is not a place or a setting; it is a group of services, individualized for their child, to support her learning needs in any context (within the regular curriculum or a special classroom). When a special education plan is set up for a child, it will specify the number of hours, the types of services, the adult-to-child ratio, and where the services will be delivered (in the regular classroom, in a special setting, and so on). In most parts of the United States, and in many other countries, a child who is performing at or close to grade level and displays relatively few challenging behaviors (for example, outbursts, aggression, interrupting) will be served in the general education setting, with appropriate supports. Special education services are delivered in the regular classroom, by the teacher and perhaps an aide, in consultation with a member of the school's special education staff. Regular classrooms, however, have a high student-to-teacher ratio, and busy teachers may not notice when the child doesn't understand something or needs help or clarification. Problems in comprehension, abstract reasoning, and organization may go unrecognized if the child has good reading and calculation skills. Teasing may not be monitored, and development of social skills may not be a focus of remediation as it might be in a special education classroom. So even children with milder or higher-functioning ASD will usually still need some special accommodations in the regular classroom to help them be successful.

To reiterate a theme from Chapter 4, *your active participation in your child's educational program is essential.* You are an expert on your child. You understand his strengths, interests, routines, triggers, and what has and has not worked for him in the past. School personnel, on the other hand, are specialists in academic policies, classroom settings and options, educational principles, and grade-appropriate curricula. The old adage "two heads are better than one" is particularly apt in this situation, so actively collaborate with your child's teachers and principal in setting up educational goals and a curriculum. Your job is a tough one, because you must walk a fine line between advocating for your child's special needs (which may be more obvious to you than to his or her teachers and the school administrators) and working *with* the school in a collegial and professional fashion. Choose your battles and be willing to compromise. This is easier said than done, we know, but it is very important to try to prevent the development of an adversarial relationship with your child's school since, in our experience, this *never* helps your child.

Special Education Options—and What Is an IEP?

Since the 1970s, federal legislation has required states to provide equal educational opportunities to all children with disabilities. In 1975, the U.S. Congress passed Public Law 94-142, which established the basic right to a "free and appropriate public education" for children with disabilities. In addition, this congressional bill mandated that schools provide a fair and unbiased evaluation to determine eligibility for services and place children in the "least restrictive" setting that could meet their educational needs. Specific special education services and goals for the child were to be listed formally in an Individualized Education Program, or IEP.

Steps in Finding the Right Program for Your Child

1. As soon as you receive the diagnosis, contact the principal of your child's school.
   - Explain the test results.
   - Ask for a referral to the school personnel who conduct eligibility determinations for special education.
2. After determining whether your child is eligible for special education, find out about different classroom options in your district.
   - Visit the different classrooms and interview the teachers.
   - Ask about the availability of certain accommodations or the willingness to provide them.
3. If your child is not eligible for special education, request an appointment with the district's "504 Coordinator."
   - Request a 504 evaluation.
   - Ask about the availability of certain accommodations or the willingness to provide them.

Parents were strongly encouraged to participate in decision making about their child's education by being part of the team that set up the IEP. Although this legislation is almost 40 years old and has undergone a number of amendments (and new names), its spirit remains strong and continues to regulate special education eligibility and delivery of services today. The current law that governs special education, the Individuals with Disabilities Education Act (or IDEA), was reauthorized by the U.S. Senate in 2004.

While these statutes grant specific educational rights to your child, it is important to understand that obtaining these rights involves a very intense process. Many stages and layers of development must be passed through on the way to putting a program into place for an individual child. Through these stages and layers, you may find that your local school is cooperative and open to new ideas, or you may find that the school has a preset agenda and is less willing to compromise. If you reach the latter point, you should be prepared to advocate for your child. It is paramount that you know your rights and responsibilities. Contact your state's department of education to get information about the special education process in your state.

In the meantime, also be aware that an ASD diagnosis (or indeed *any* psychological or psychiatric diagnosis) does *not* guarantee that your child will qualify for special education services. Eligibility is determined by examining the impact of the condition on your child's academic skills and other areas of functioning in the school setting. Different states implement the federal guidelines in different manners. After obtaining a diagnosis, parents should take the diagnostic report (or ask that it be sent) to their child's school and request an evaluation to assess her educational needs. It is possible that the results of this evaluation will indicate that your child does not qualify for special education services. If so, don't lose heart—there are other options for receiving support in the school, which are discussed in a later section on classroom accommodations and 504 Plans.

If your child does prove eligible for special education, then an IEP will be prepared, with much input from you. The IEP is best thought of as a contract between parents and schools that outlines what the team agrees is an appropriate education for the child, how and where the services will be delivered, and how it will be evaluated to see if it is working. The IDEA law mandates that a "team" develop, review, and revise the IEP. The IEP team consists of:

1. A school representative (other than teachers) qualified to offer or supervise special education services (if your district has an autism specialist, she may serve in this role; alternate possibilities include the director of special education or another school administrator).
2. The child's regular and special education teachers.
3. Other school personnel providing services to the child (for example, occupational and/or speech therapists).

4. Parents.
5. The child, when possible and if age-appropriate.

As a member of the IEP team, you have some choices and some power in the decision-making process, more so than you may be accustomed to with your children without ASD. If there is something you think your child needs at school (such as language services, social skills training, help with goal setting and organization, reading comprehension tutoring, an aide), your best recourse is to get it put in the IEP. Keep in mind, too, that you can ask to include on the team anyone with special knowledge or expertise concerning the needs of your child.

Know your legal rights. For example, you do not need to sign the IEP until you agree that it provides what you think your child needs and the law promises you. Equally important, however, is understanding that the law says your child is entitled to an *appropriate* education, not the *best* education. Just as with regular education, parents may choose to "purchase" what they perceive to be the *best* education for their child through a private school. That said, keep in mind that the educational plan must be individualized— that is, specifically tailored to meet the unique needs of your child. This means that the school must develop a unique plan for each student, regardless of what the school offers other children.

What happens if you disagree with your school over the appropriate/best distinction? For example, sometimes parents think that a particular service is *appropriate* for their child with ASD and therefore should be funded by the school system, but school personnel see this service as *the best* technique, and therefore not something the school is obligated to provide. In our experience, a combination of persistence and willingness to negotiate will often get parents fairly close to what they desire in the IEP. If, however, after a series of negotiations with the school, you still feel the program being offered by the school is not appropriate, you can contact your state education department to find out what alternatives are available. The federal government has mandated that every state have an agency designated to help parents get through the special education process.

IEPs contain specific goals and objectives for your child's education. A *goal* is a general desired change in your child's learning, skills, or behaviors, while an *objective* is the specific definition of that change and how it will be measured. Goals are usually broader and longer term (perhaps set annually), while objectives are shorter-term benchmarks for determining whether appropriate progress toward the goal is being made. For example, an IEP goal might be "to increase reading comprehension," while a corresponding objective would be "to answer questions about a paragraph accurately 75% of the time." It is important to choose IEP goals and objectives that are both meaningful and realistic. You want the skills specified to be ones that are important to your child's functionality, independence, and later success, while also being attainable. If IEP objectives are set too high, it will appear that your child is "failing" when in fact she is really straining to meet an inappropriate skill level. If the objective is set too low, your child may not be challenged appropriately and therefore not receive the level of intervention that she could benefit from. And remember that an IEP is not immutable: at any time, any member of the IEP team (including you as parents) can ask that the IEP be reviewed and revised. This is typically done at least annually and more often if necessary. If objectives are being met at an unanticipated pace or not met at all or if new diagnostic or evaluation results are obtained, then a meeting of the IEP team is warranted.

In addition to specific goals and objectives, IEPs contain a list of related services that will be provided to your child in the school setting, such as speech–language therapy, occupational therapy, adaptive physical education, or social skills training. Some children with ASD need one-on-one instruction for certain academic tasks or during certain activities (for example, groups) when their behavior or understanding may limit their ability to benefit otherwise from the instruction. In such cases, a request for an aide can be made in the IEP. An aide can be full- or part-time and can be assigned to an individual student or shared among a few students who would all benefit from smaller group learning. Aides can be extremely valuable, but they are usually paraprofessionals without any advanced degrees (or perhaps even formal training). Therefore, it is important to request that your aide either have prior experience or receive specific training in both standard educational principles and best practices for students with ASD. It is also important to ensure that your child's aide gives him chances to "practice" the skills without always jumping in to help. Too much one-to-one assistance can be as bad as too little. Specifically, it may make your child overly dependent on prompts from an adult and therefore may reduce the child's initiative and ability to function independently. Aides need to know how to provide subtle structure without eliminating chances for the child to interact, practice, and try, before offering more help.

Classroom Options

Children can receive special education services in a self-contained classroom—one whose members all have difficulties of some type and who are all receiving special education—or in regular classrooms, partially or even primarily. Over the last few decades, across the United States and many other parts of the world, there has been a strong movement toward "inclusion" of children with ASD, at all levels of functioning, in regular education. This means that, whenever possible, the child's education, including services specified in her IEP, are provided in regular classrooms, by a regular education teacher, in collaboration with special education staff. This has the benefit of surrounding the child with typically developing peers and exposing the child to appropriate behavior and good models of age-typical communication and interpersonal relationships. In fact, one basic principle within special education legislation is that all children with disabilities should be educated in the "least restrictive environment" (this principle is often nick-

named "LRE" by school staff), alongside children who are not disabled, and that putting children in self-contained classes should be
minimized. The child may be "pulled out" of the regular classroom
only for special services like occupational therapy, and even then
these may be delivered in a small-group format, with other children. "LRE" is part of federal law, so school personnel will always
start by offering your child the least restrictive educational setting,
with appropriate supports. If there is evidence that her needs are
not being met in such a setting, then the IEP team can meet and
add more services or change the setting in which the services are
delivered, as needed.

Public or Private School?

Parents sometimes turn to private schools when they feel that their
child's unique needs can't be met by the public school options in
their region. Private schools may seem to have a clear advantage
since most offer substantially smaller class sizes and more individualized instruction than public schools. But there are other factors
to consider. Perhaps the most important is that private schools are
not governed by the federal laws that mandate a "free and appropriate" public education. Obviously, private schooling is not free,
and private schools are not required to provide "appropriate" services. So keep in mind that a move to a private school will involve
relinquishing your legal right to these services.

Another consideration, however, is the uniformity and homo-
geneity of the school. In some private schools there is so little
diversity and the student body is so geared toward high achievement that the child with ASD stands out far more than in a public
school. In some private schools, it can be so much harder to fit in
that it is not worth the other benefits the setting might offer.

Finally, money is often an issue. Many families need to choose
among a variety of therapeutic options and must constantly weigh
the costs against the benefits. Will this money be better spent else-

where? If we choose this private school, will we need to give up speech therapy or social skills training? This is another example of the need to "choose your battles."

· There are private schools that will agree to provide educational accommodations appropriate for children with ASD and some that even specialize in such accommodations. In this case such a school may be a good setting for your child. If you do find a special school of this type, be sure that it provides opportunities for inclusion and education with nondisabled students as well. The principle of the "least restrictive environment" is not just legal policy but is also good for your child's social development.

Classroom Accommodations—and What Is a 504 Plan?

As mentioned above, all is not lost if your child does not qualify for special education and an IEP. The Federal Rehabilitation Act of 1973 is a law that protects the civil and constitutional rights of people with disabilities. Section 504 of this law (since renamed the Americans with Disabilities Act, or ADA) mandates access to a free and appropriate public education for all people with disabilities. Disabilities are broadly defined in this legislation (more broadly than in IDEA, the special education law) as any limit in any major life activity, including "learning." At first, this law was interpreted as an obligation to provide *physical* access to education for people with disabilities (for example, curb cuts and elevators for students in wheelchairs, sign language interpreters for deaf students, and the like). More recently, however, the meaning of "access" to an appropriate education has been expanded. Section 504 has increasingly been used to secure services for children with disabilities who don't qualify for special education but still have educational needs (or, in the language of the law, "limits in learning"). All school districts have a designated "504 coordinator" who helps put together services for children qualified under Section 504. In brief, a "504 Plan" is a written document that lays out a variety of modifications that a child needs to be successful in a regular education environment. Usually these accommodations are somewhat less time-consuming and require less intensive intervention and fewer trained staff to implement them than those provided via an IEP. The downside to 504 Plans (relative to IEPs) is that there is no federal funding to implement them; thus, whatever you ask your school to provide in a 504 Plan must be done with the school's existing funds or at no additional cost. In the following sections, we outline a variety of interventions and accommodations that can be added to a 504 Plan to help your child succeed (not just survive) in school, despite the learning and/or behavioral difficulties of ASD. It is also worth mentioning that these very same accommodations can be part of an IEP (in other words, 504 goals are not mutually exclusive of IEP goals) if your child qualifies for special education under IDEA.

Teacher and Classroom Characteristics

One of the most important ingredients in a successful school program is the teacher—specifically, the teacher's level of flexibility, open-mindedness, positive attitude, sense of humor, and willingness to try new things. Teachers who appreciate diversity, accept students as they are, and enjoy the uniqueness of those with ASD are particularly valuable. You may find these qualities in teachers in regular classrooms, self-contained special education classrooms, or private schools. The following characteristics are often seen in the classrooms of teachers who have successfully served children with high-functioning ASD (and with other special needs):

- Consistent routines and rules
- Consistent places that assignment materials are kept and assignments are collected
- A posted classroom schedule
- Use of clear, simple, unambiguous language
- Provision of written instructions (such as directions written on the chalkboard)

- Preferential desk placement near the teacher and away from distractions, such as windows or corridors
- A special work station when noise or other distractions disrupt work
- Allocation of sufficient time for instructions, repetition of instructions, and individual student assistance
- Frequent monitoring of student work pace and work product
- Directing of questions toward the students to see that they understand the work and are attending
- Immediate feedback on performance, including reinforcement for both effort and productivity

Some school districts will allow parents to visit several classrooms and hand-pick a teacher and classroom that possess these qualities, whether it is in the child's neighborhood school or not. And many teachers who do not already do these things will be willing to if asked. Many of these things will benefit all students in the class and are not particularly time-consuming for the teacher. They are prime examples of the kinds of modifications that can be listed in your child's 504 Plan or IEP.

A wide variety of additional accommodations that may help your child can be added to a 504 Plan or an IEP. Some of these are, in contrast to the preceding list, more work for a teacher who may already be juggling a large class and be terribly overworked. Some of these accommodations may draw unwanted attention to your child and make him stand out in a way that turns out to be unacceptable to you or the teachers. Sometimes school personnel worry that providing a service to one child will open the floodgates to similar requests for other children, so they resist your request for the accommodation. Also remember that there is no extra funding coming to your school to pay for the modifications listed in a 504 Plan. For all these reasons, it is important to choose judiciously from the ideas presented below and ask specifically for those that you feel will truly be helpful for your child.

Workload

You may find that your child has hours of homework each evening, perhaps much more than other students in the class. This may be due to her working slowly and inefficiently as a result of being preoccupied by special interests or distracted by details, as well as to the poorly developed concept of time so often seen in children with ASD. This often places a large burden on parents, because your child will likely need a great deal of structure and supervision from you to finish this homework. We saw a couple in our clinic who were so stressed by their son's hours of homework and his resistance to completing it that it created terrible friction between them and eventually (combined with other stresses) led to their divorce. If your situation is in any way similar, even if not quite so extreme, you may want to ask your child's teacher to consider some of the following options for managing time.

If your child seems unaware of passing time, then an intervention as simple as providing a kitchen timer or watch with an alarm can be used to help your child monitor her work pace. These devices provide concrete cues for the beginning and end of each work activity, as well as advance warnings of deadlines. Another option that may be necessary is decreasing your child's workload. Perhaps the number of problems required could be reduced (for example, your child must complete 10 math problems instead of the 20 that classmates must finish) or the assignment shortened (writing one versus four paragraphs on a particular topic). If your child can still learn a concept without doing quite so many problems, this may be a possibility. Another option is to have less information on a page so that the amount of work *appears* less, even if it truly is not. A child faced with one page of 10 math problems may be overwhelmed, but the same child who faces a few pages of less dense problems (perhaps three per page) may find the work manageable. When your child reaches junior and senior high school and perhaps college, an additional version of this principle is to limit the number of courses taken. It may be best for the student to enroll in two to three classes per semester, instead of the usual four or five, especially when the classes are time-consuming or difficult. We also recommend enrolling in small classes, where the amount of attention from the professor may be greater. Or your child may want to choose less popular classes (we know a college student with ASD who chose to take Russian instead of Spanish), where class size may be smaller and professors may be highly motivated to retain students. It is more important for your child to have a successful experience than to follow a typical schedule. You may also want to ask that certain curriculum requirements be waived, especially those that prove difficult for many people with ASD, like foreign language classes.

Visual Strategies

As we've highlighted throughout this book, children and adolescents with ASD are often visual learners. Thus, providing as much visual input and structure as possible will help most students with ASD. For example, teachers could be asked to write instructions they give to the whole class on the chalkboard, so that if your child is not paying attention for a moment or cannot process the verbal instructions quickly, he has a record and reminder of what to do. The teacher might also provide your child with individual instructions, in the form of a written prompt or reminder on an index card that can be taped to his desk. Another example of providing visual structure is to show your child a model of the final goal or completed product. It is often easier to work toward the conclusion when the child can *see* what he is supposed to be doing than if the end product is abstract or otherwise intangible.

Executive Function Help

Several strategies can be used to compensate for organization and planning difficulties, also called *executive function problems*, that your child may demonstrate. One is a *weekly homework log* that is sent from school to home and back, keeping all parties informed of work due and progress on it. A description of the homework and the due date are entered in the log by your child, often with the teacher's help. Teachers may need to check that your child has all homework and associated materials before leaving school. Parents can then enter their initials in the log to indicate that their child has worked on the assignment at home, and teachers can sign off when it has been turned in. Teachers can indicate grades received as well as the number of times that homework was not completed on time. You may also want to request that teachers give your child advance warning of upcoming due dates, even before other students in the class, so that she has extra time to complete the assignment.

Assignment checklists can be used to help break large, often overwhelming, tasks into manageable units. For example, an assignment checklist might contain information about how to get started ("Begin with question 7 on page 4"), what to do (every other item, for example), how to recognize when the task is complete ("Finish 10 problems"), where to store or hand in the completed product (for example, a backpack near the door), and a reminder to clean up. For larger assignments, timelines might be supplied along with a list of subgoals. For example, if your child has a book report due at the end of the month, you or the teacher could not only break this large goal into its smaller objectives (visit library, choose book, read book, outline main ideas, and so on), but assign due dates for each of these subgoals. Otherwise, your child may start the process only a day or two in advance since he hasn't realized the length of time that each of the smaller goals will require. It is also helpful to provide a list of materials needed for each assignment (perhaps a calculator, specific assignment sheet, the correct book, a writing implement). While this may seem obvious, one of the most common reasons that students with ASD fail to complete work is that they don't have the appropriate materials ready when they sit down to work.

Day planners, simplified versions of the kind that many adults use, can also help organize your child. All events with a designated time should be entered in the planner, including, for example, time to wake up, eat breakfast, and get to the bus stop; time for major school activities and after-school appointments; and times for dinner, homework, relaxation, and bed. Children enjoy it when an empty box is placed next to each item, to be filled with a check mark or sticker once the activity has been completed. This provides a visual concrete cue identifying completed and upcoming events. Since day planners are widely used and do not make the child stand out from peers, they tend to be well accepted. It may also be helpful for parents to adopt a day planner themselves, modeling its use for their child. Also, including things your child likes or considers special, such as calculators, favorite writing implements, money, or trading cards, in a pouch in the day planner can increase its relevance and worth, reducing the likelihood that it will be "forgotten" at home or school. Once your child is older, and perhaps has access to her own electronics (phone or tablet), she will have the skills necessary to begin using the calendar provided on such devices.

"To do" lists can be included in the day planner for tasks that need to get done but do not have specific designated times (errands, telephone calls, chores, and so on). You'll need to teach your child to cross out items as they are completed, and then each evening to transfer items that have yet to be finished to the next day's list. Items on the list can be prioritized with a numbering or color-coding system.

Help–Seeking Routines

Because of their social challenges and their difficulty initiating interactions, students with ASD often do not ask for help when they need it. Therefore, it is important for teachers to be on the lookout for the need for help, to check in with your child periodically to monitor work, and to create signals or other routines that your child can use to indicate the need for help. Sometimes this can be as simple as teaching the child to raise his hand. If a child is particularly self-conscious and unlikely to call attention to himself in this way, however, the teacher could supply a specific but unobtrusive behavior that the child could use to signal the need for help—perhaps turning sideways, with feet toward the aisle rather than directly under the desk, or placing a special object on the desktop.

Group Learning.

Social difficulties can also present an obstacle to group work for the child with ASD. Since the 1990s, the educational principle of collaborative learning has been prominent in American schools. Children work in groups to complete a common product. The goal of this type of instruction is learning to work together, to negotiate, and to help one another. It is not sufficient for each child to focus on her individual goal or part of the task; one weak link, and the whole project will receive a lower grade. This practice appears to have many obvious educational and less tangible social benefits. However, as you might imagine, this kind of work is very hard for the child with ASD. At the worst, it can mean that your child does not learn particular concepts because the learning process so much depends on social skills. If so, you may find it necessary to request another learning format (such as individual assignments) for your child. On the other hand, if your child shows some ability to participate in group exercises, they can be great social opportunities.

Difficulties can also arise when students are expected to work in self-chosen pairs or teams. It can be exceedingly painful to be the only one "not picked," a not uncommon situation for students with ASD. In such circumstances, parents can encourage teachers to draw numbers or use some other means of pairing off in classes.

Handwriting Alternatives

Many people with ASD have poor handwriting. It can be very difficult to read, as well as slow and laborious to produce. This often results in anxiety, resistance to activities that involve hand-writing, and even some of the challenging behaviors we described in the last chapter. To alleviate some of these problems, you can ask that your child's teacher provide extra time for and/or shorten written assignments. Also, it's important that your child be graded on content, not the neatness or legibility of his or her handwriting. You can also ask your child's teacher to allow him or her to submit work in an alternative form (typed on a computer, audio-recorded, dictated to a peer or parent), with the exception of those tasks that were designed specifically to promote and develop hand-writing. Many schools now provide access to laptop computers or to keyboards that are connected to a central classroom computer and printer.

Labored handwriting makes note taking difficult for students with ASD (as does their slower auditory processing and their tendency to become preoccupied with details and special interests). It is very helpful if teachers give a copy of their notes or an outline of the class discussion to students with ASD (preferably before-hand), so that they can listen to lectures and concentrate on what the teacher adds while speaking, without the frustration of taking notes. Another possibility is asking that a peer provide copies of his notes to the child or teen with ASD. Permitting audio recording of lectures is another method to assist with note taking. Similarly, copying from the chalkboard can be a challenge (due not only to writing problems but also to the child's need to constantly switch back and forth between two tasks: reading and writing). Access to teacher or classmate notes will significantly reduce this problem too. Some parents worry that these accommodations will place an unnecessary spotlight on their child. In our experience, however, these academic modifications can make your child fit in better and in the long run actually reduce the spotlight on your child. At the college level, it is the rule rather than the exception that teachers provide lecture outlines to students, so you might encourage your child's teachers to provide the notes to everyone in the class, not just the student with ASD.

Test Taking

Test taking is another academic activity that often presents special challenges to the child with ASD, even the most high-functioning among them, due to the combination of time management, handwriting, anxiety, and executive function problems. The student could be permitted to take exams in an alternative format (for example, orally, or by using a fill-in-the-blanks written format), to have extra time for tests, and to take them in a quiet room, alone, or with a teacher or aide present to provide structure and motivation, interpret questions, and manage time.

Alberto is an 11-year-old diagnosed with ASD. He is educated within regular classrooms. In science class they were learning about species' classification, a topic that Alberto particularly enjoyed and was good at—his excellent memory helped him learn the Latin names and categories easily. His mother was therefore quite surprised when he brought home a test on animal classification with a large red F on the top. When she went in to talk to the science teacher, she found that the format of the test was very different from other tests, as well as from how Alberto and his classmates had learned and studied the material. Specifically, the teacher had given students a page of animal names that they were supposed to cut out and then arrange on a chart according to their species. While Alberto knew every name and classification by heart, he was not able to flexibly apply this knowledge to this new format. His mother demonstrated for the teacher how Alberto could fill in the blanks or answer short questions about every animal on the chart and how, in fact, he could even complete the chart once his mother explained the task to him and provided one example. She then requested a new IEP meeting and had it written formally into Alberto's IEP that he be allowed to take tests for all his classes in the resource room, where the resource teacher could monitor his work and provide assistance and clarification when necessary. In addition, it was included in Alberto's IEP that his tests follow a standard format (specifically, fill-in-the-blank and short-answer questions). His mother and the resource teacher were also promised that they would be given advance notice of any test that would, of necessity, follow a different format so that they could teach Alberto how to respond in a different way and be sure he understood what was asked of him.

Comprehension and Abstraction Skills

Some high-functioning children with ASD will not exhibit any academic problems in their first few years of school. Parents may be told that the child is academically on a par with the other children or perhaps even more advanced than classmates in some areas. For some children, this advantage dwindles with time and they begin to fall behind classmates as the grades advance. This usually occurs because the concepts taught in school become progressively more abstract and require more interpretation, integration, and generalization than they did in lower grades. Thus, the strengths of most children with ASD described in Chapter 5, such as memory and visualization, are highlighted in early grades but are progressively less required as the years go by. Conversely, the comprehension and abstraction skills that seem to be integral parts of the cognitive deficit profile of ASD are increasingly required. What can be done to help your child with these kinds of skills?

Most of the answers to this question have already been provided somewhere in this chapter: make concepts as concrete and visual as possible, organize the work in advance, and use special interests or skills when you can. At the risk of some redundancy, we will provide some specific examples of how to use these principles to compensate for weaknesses in reading comprehension and math concepts.

Reading Comprehension. Capitalizing on the rule-following strength of ASD, teachers and parents can teach rules for understanding stories. Especially in elementary grades, most stories have a common structure that includes four typical elements: (1) who, (2) did what, (3) and then, (4) the end. That is, someone (the "who" of the story) does or is involved in something (the "what"), which is followed by some resolution of the situation, and then an ending. Teachers can underline these elements in a story or highlight them in color-coded ink in advance. They can provide a list of questions in the same color ink, thus tapping into visual strengths to improve comprehension. Or they can ask students to generate alternate but plausible endings to the story or paraphrase the main points by retelling the story in their own words (pictures or a visual flowchart can be used to make this exercise as concrete as possible). Teachers need to be alert for rote or memorized responses that come straight from the story without true understanding (such as echoing sentences rather than restating ideas in the child's own words). Additional elements of story grammar, such as the location or setting ("where") and the reasons, intentions, or motives of characters ("why"), can be added as the child is able to handle them. But add the last item with care. It is often difficult for children with ASD to judge the underlying human motives and interpersonal dynamics of a situation, so they may be able to get a reasonable handle on the rest of the story's structure, only to be stymied by this one element.

Alex, a 16-year-old with ASD, explained why he was failing 11th-grade English. "My teachers," he said, "are always asking me questions that they know the answers to, but I don't. Even when I try to figure out *why* someone did something in *The Scarlet Letter*, it's never the reason the teacher thinks they did it. I just have different ideas about things than they do. I especially hate to speculate why someone else did something. I can only say why I did something." Alex was fascinated with animals, especially endangered species, and was much better able to answer "why" questions about these topics than about Hester Prynne.

Math. As with reading (and much else in this chapter), improving comprehension of math concepts boils down to making the abstract concrete and visual. Whenever possible, students with ASD should be allowed to use manipulative materials (rods, tokens, beans, and the like) to stand in for abstract concepts like addition, subtraction, multiplication, and division. They can be allowed to act out or draw pictures to represent the components in word problems. Critical aspects of word problems can be highlighted or color-coded in advance by teachers so that the student will recognize information pertaining to which mathematical operation should be performed or which variables should be attended to. To see how word problems correspond to mathematical calculations, students can make up their own word problems revolving around their special interests. For example, "7–5" becomes "If you had seven trains and lost five of them, how many would you have left?" There should be explicit practice generalizing math skills to real-life situations, as this often does not happen naturally. Toward that end, fractions can be practiced by learning to follow recipes, subtraction can be illustrated by calculating whether the appropriate amount of change has been received back from a fast-food purchase, and money concepts can be taught using catalogs of favorite items and menus from favorite restaurants.

Behavioral Issues

It may also be necessary for your school to set up a behavior plan or contract to deal with nonacademic challenging behaviors your child may demonstrate in school (such as interrupting, distracting others, constantly talking about topics of special interest, and aggression) that influence her education. Many of the behavioral interventions discussed in Chapters 4 and 6 can be helpful in the school setting, including frequently reinforcing desired behavior (perhaps using tokens or other systems), ignoring minor misbehavior, teaching the child self-management techniques, performing a thorough analysis of the function of the problem behavior, and supplying the child with alternative, more acceptable behaviors to achieve the same goals. Many teachers are trained in these techniques and use them with all their students, not just those with ASD.

Transitions

Each new school year brings anxiety for both parent and child. The transition between elementary and middle school is often a particularly scary time, because your child will now have to negotiate multiple teachers and classrooms. You may be able to alleviate some of this anxiety by planning a visit to the new school at the end of the summer to explore the building and begin to learn the locations of classrooms, locker, lunchroom, and bus stop. Your child may also need to practice his locker combination. You can ask the school to provide this in advance and then buy an inexpensive lock for home practice (it won't open, of course, to the same combination as the one at school, but your child can memorize the numbers and practice turning the dial in the appropriate directions). It may also be useful to ask school personnel to consider the physical layout of the building when scheduling your child's classes. They may be able to assign a locker that is relatively close to the different rooms or choose classes that happen to meet near each other, thus minimizing your child's travel time and the chance for confusion or tardiness. Provision of a school map with classrooms highlighted and numbered in the order in which the courses are scheduled can also be a useful visual tool.

Making transitions between teachers and negotiating their individual expectations and standards can also be difficult for the student with ASD. One way to minimize this problem is to designate a supportive, central contact person such as a school counselor or resource teacher, who helps coordinate services, monitor progress, schedule meetings, and provide comfort and support to the child when needed. Ask to have such a coordinator designated as part of the IEP or 504 Plan. If your school has an autism team, choose someone from this team. It is often best if this "go-to" person is someone other than a classroom teacher, because negotiating among the needs of the child, the desires of parents, the style of the teacher, and the constraints of the educational system can be very tricky.

Some Concluding Thoughts

Some of the problems described in this chapter could be eliminated if school personnel were educated regarding the learning style of students with ASD. This education may start when you alert the school about your child's diagnosis. Some parents fear that sharing diagnostic information with educators will negatively "label" their son or daughter, resulting in substandard education or inappropriate reduction of academic and behavioral expectations. In our experience, this is rarely the case. In fact, as this chapter should make clear, a wide variety of special services, therapies, and accommodations can be provided in the school, at no cost to you or your family, that will help your child succeed in school. To access such services, however, you must make the specific nature of your child's educational needs known. This includes sharing diagnostic information and other test results that may be relevant. It may also mean steering interested educators and administrators to resources and information about ASD. The Resources at the back of this book include sources specific to the educational needs of students with ASD that may be helpful to share with school personnel.

An important consideration is that your child's academic curriculum address functional and adaptive skills that she will need to be successful in later life. One of the most important outcomes of school for children and adolescents with mild ASD is establishing good work habits, a positive self-concept, and independent living skills. This may mean that there will need to be considerable flexibility in designing your child's curriculum and an understanding that it may not follow the standard curriculum. Parents and teachers need to constantly ask, "Does this contribute to this child's long-term goals?" This is vastly more important than following a typical curriculum outline or worrying about the number of credits needed to graduate.

Finally, in keeping with a central theme of this book, it is always important to capitalize on your child's strengths to compensate for academic difficulties or areas of weakness in school. Many examples are already woven throughout this chapter. For example, supplementing oral directions with visual aids is a way to use your child's well-developed visualization skills to make up for one of his weaker skills. Similarly, giving your child written directions or written rules is a way to use his reading skills to maintain focus and teach more appropriate behavior. Your child's special interests can be used to motivate him in the classroom.

Joseph's teacher was considering using his interest in geography to counteract his growing boredom and disinterest in other academic subjects. His parents proposed that subjects and skills taught to Joseph incorporate something related to geography whenever possible. For example, when the class was learning to make timelines in history, his parents asked the teacher to allow Joseph to make a timeline of explorers and their discoveries of different parts of the world. In science, when the rest of the class learned about the geology of California, Joseph was allowed to learn about the geology of his favorite country at the time, Brazil. In math, Joseph's teacher devised simple problems involving the mileage between different cities in California. And during reading, he let Joseph read any book he chose, rather than the one the class was reading together. In this way, his teachers and parents made positive use of his intense focus on geography, motivating him to work and rescuing his plummeting grades in all academic subjects. After seeing the success of this relatively simple intervention, Joseph's teacher added a geography unit for the whole class, even though it was not typically part of the third grade curriculum, and allowed Joseph to act as the "assistant teacher" during the module. He also asked Joseph to go to younger classrooms to read to children. This "special job" made Joseph feel important and good about some of his abilities, despite the teasing and other failures he was also experiencing at school. Helping others is often a very successful way to build self-esteem and self-efficacy.

Another way to use your child's talents to promote school success is to involve her in any school clubs or activities that use those talents or involve those special interests. Enroll your daughter in the computer club or the reading club. If your school doesn't have one already, volunteer to organize and run it. If your child has a natural talent for spelling, encourage her to participate in spelling bees. These activities will help integrate your child into the life of the school and help her feel like part of the school community rather than a peripheral member. Many other social issues raise their heads in the school setting as well—one of the most painful for parents is the teasing or bullying of their beloved son or daughter. It is to these tender issues that we turn our attention next, in Chapter 8.

8

The Social World of Children and Adolescents with High-Functioning Autism Spectrum Disorder

"Hello, Friend—Now Go Away"

Everyone diagnosed with ASD has trouble with social interchanges, specifically with what we call *reciprocity,* the back-and-forth interactions that make up all social encounters. In the very remote, nonverbal children who have the most severe symptoms of ASD, reciprocity difficulties are obvious. In high-functioning children and adolescents with ASD, however, reciprocity problems may be more subtle. Parents often describe a feeling of one-sidedness in interactions with their child. Sometimes parents feel as if they must carry the whole relationship, supporting and scaffolding the interaction to establish some meaningful connection. If they don't start the conversation or ask the specific questions, the child may have very little to say or appear totally content on his own. Other parents describe their child as having his own agenda: the child either tells the parents what to do or talks on and on without paying much attention to the parents or altering his behavior in response to what the parents say or do.

When Seth starts talking about the stock market or the national debt, there is no stopping him. During dinner, he likes to tell his parents about the NASDAQ's performance that day. After repeated attempts to introduce other topics at the dinner table, his exasperated parents find themselves ignoring Seth when he talks about finances and carrying on their own conversation. They aren't sure whether to be worried or relieved that Seth barely seems to notice that they aren't paying attention and keeps talking. If they make a comment or try to add any relevant information, Seth pauses politely but then takes up where he left off, as if his parents hadn't said a word. His parents do consider this a small success, since just a year earlier Seth would become extremely upset whenever anyone made a comment and feel compelled to start anew, repeating every single thing he had said prior to the point of "interruption."

Social reciprocity problems may be even more evident with peers. Children and teens with ASD are often described as "on the periphery." They can be seen walking around the perimeter of the playground, uninvolved and seemingly uninterested in the boisterous play going on around them. They may demonstrate a strong need for control and insist that other kids follow their own rules. If peers balk at this, the child with ASD may complain or express sadness because "other kids don't want to play what I want to play," but show little ability or motivation to negotiate or compromise.

Seth's parents often got reports from his teacher that Seth was "bossy" with other kids. They asked the school psychologist to observe Seth on the playground to collect some examples of this behavior, so that they would be able to work with him at home using specific situations and examples from the school day. The psychologist told them that Seth spent most of recess walking around the playground fence, talking to himself under his breath. When other children called out to him, Seth usually didn't seem to notice. Occasionally, he would reluctantly

join games in progress. During the psychologist's observation, Seth accepted an invitation to play freeze-tag but then
insisted that no one touch him and that he be allowed to be
"it" immediately. He protested loudly and tried to hit the child
who tagged him out. Seth eventually went back to the fence,
where he began to drag a stick against it as he circled the playground's edge, far from the other children.

In structured settings, such as school or scout groups, some
children or teens with ASD may interact with other kids and even
feel a bond with some of them, but few pursue these relationships
outside these settings. For the few individuals with ASD who do
seek out other children outside prearranged situations, often there
is still a relative lack of depth in the relationship. It may not be
fully mutual, with one person being more committed to and interested in the relationship than the other. The relationship may be
limited in focus, revolving primarily around a shared interest—for
example, the kids may play video games side by side, but don't
do anything else together. Or the friendship may not involve the
same level of intimacy (for example, sharing secrets and feelings,
relying on each other for support or help) as expected for a child
of that age. Research studies show that many children with high-
functioning ASD have a very limited concept of friendship. When
asked what it means to be a friend, they give simple and concrete
explanations ("someone who is nice to you" or "you play with
them") and are much less likely than other children of the same
age to mention qualities such as companionship, affection, selectivity, and trust.

Derrick, a young boy with ASD, volunteered that he had
many friends but then added poignantly, "Some of them are
mean to me." Upon further questioning, it came out that Derrick considered anyone in his class whose name he knew to
be his friend. Like many children with ASD, Derrick was very
vulnerable to teasing because of his social naivete and unusual
style of relating to others. He recounted how earlier that day

a classmate had given him a piece of candy; after he'd taken a taste, the child "informed" Derrick that the candy had "drugs" in it. Derrick spent the rest of the school day worried and crying.

How children and adolescents with ASD react to their lack of friends and to peer rejection varies. Some desperately desire friends and feel left out and lonely. Others seem quite content; they either don't notice or don't care that they have no friends—they are truly "loners" at heart. Still others vary at different ages, in different settings, or from hour to hour, vacillating between feelings of loneliness and taking pleasure in solitude. Some adults in our social support group articulately describe a yearning for contact with others, but then only limited tolerance for brief interactions (summarized in one Internet chat room as "Hello, friend—now go away").

Social reciprocity problems are also evident in conversation. There may be very little back-and-forth, with domination by the person with ASD, who does not pick up on cues from the other person that he or she has something to say (as with Seth). The child with high-functioning ASD may not ask questions of others, particularly about their opinions, feelings, and experiences. The child may have difficulty keeping conversations going, particularly when direct questions are not posed.

Seth was playing on the sidewalk in front of his house with some action figures. A neighbor boy of approximately the same age came up and asked Seth where he had gotten the figures. Seth replied, "Disneyland," without looking up. The boy said excitedly, "Oh, I've been to Disneyland too!" Seth said nothing and the boy eventually walked away.

Many people with ASD ask questions when they need to find out something but are much less comfortable making comments or "small talk." In fact they may have trouble with social chat and may rarely talk purely for social purposes.

Clint was in an elevator riding up to the fourth floor of the building in which his social support group took place. The group's therapist got in on level 2 and smiled at Clint. Last week's discussion in group had been about making small talk. One of the specific situations they had role-played was what to say during a brief interaction on an elevator. A few topics had been mentioned: perhaps the weather or the traffic. Clint decided to try something new. He said to the therapist, looking him directly in the eyes as he'd learned, "Gee, what's that terrible smell?" The therapist smiled politely, shrugged, and said, "I'm not sure. How was your drive down today?" Clint persisted, saying, "Boy, something really smells bad in here!"

John, another young man in the social support group, made this comment after a group discussion about conversation. "I know there is something called 'reciprocity.' I've heard of it. I know what the word means. I know it exists. I just don't understand it. I can't even identify it when it's happening. It's much like humans might feel about echolocation [of bats— this young man's interest]. We know echolocation exists. We just can't hear it, nor would we know how to understand it if it was within our auditory range. That's how reciprocity is for me."

Kids with ASD tend not to use the same kind of social body language that others use. Their eye contact may be limited, they may not smile at the other person, their posture may not convey interest and attention, and they may not use socially encouraging gestures such as nodding. All of this can give the impression that the person with ASD is not truly engaged in the conversation, is not listening, or is bored. Other problems sometimes seen in ASD, such as aggression or an overly blunt communication style (sometimes interpreted as rude or offensive, although it is unintentional), can also pose a threat to social relationships. Even the special interests of individuals with ASD contribute to poor reciprocity because they are so focused and idiosyncratic that they are difficult for others to share (or the child doesn't actually *want* to share them, as with Seth). And there is very strong research documentation, in addition to many descriptions from parents, of lack of empathy and difficulty taking others' perspectives. All in all, kids with ASD often seem very self-centered. Although there is no intent to be selfish, and there is no malice behind their behavior, their social shortcomings can have a wide-ranging negative impact on their lives: in their relationships, on their academic and occupational success, and elsewhere.

Naturally, then, as parents you want to help your child or teenager learn to be a social creature in our social world. But how? If your son wants friends but can't make them, how can you help? What can his teachers do? What can you expect from a therapist? If your daughter seems to have little interest in friends, but needs to work on social behaviors so that she can someday live independently and keep a job, where can you turn for help? Strategies for improving social reciprocity in kids with high-functioning ASD follow.

Strategies for Improving Children's Social Behavior

Social skills can be taught in many different settings. The traditional arena is in a school or clinic, through an organized social skills group. However, as you shall see in this chapter, there are a variety of other places where and times when you can help your child acquire critical social skills: at home, around the neighborhood, and in nontherapeutic group settings (for example, scouts). Many of the principles and techniques used in typical therapeutic groups can be used by parents at home. In fact, social skills groups are much more beneficial if supplemented by follow-up at home. So whether your child attends such a group or not, it will be important for you to know what you can do outside the clinic to reinforce more appropriate social behavior too.

What Your Child's Therapist Can Offer

Group Social Skills Training

Your family may have adapted to your child's social deficits, and therefore you might not consider the problem an enormous one at home in your daily activities. But social difficulties tend to be more pronounced in groups and with peers. So social problems may in fact be fairly significant for your child at school, at the local playground, or in a scout troop. We know that people with ASD have trouble generalizing from one situation to another, so it's important to teach social skills in settings that are similar to those in which the children experience difficulty. When teaching social behavior to a child with high-functioning ASD, the therapist or teacher may be impressed by how fast the child learns new skills, only to be surprised later at how poorly these skills are applied, in real-world settings, with peers. Thus, teaching in a group context is essential.

Formal instruction, with specific skills taught sequentially, is also important. Most parents are not equipped to deliver this type of instruction, so you will probably have to look for a group at an outpatient clinic or school, where the therapy will be delivered by a therapist or teacher. This does not mean, however, that you're not part of the process. As managers of your child's care, you should think of yourselves as consumers of the social skills training that teachers and therapists can offer your child. If the group training offered to your child diverges substantially from what we describe here, in ways that seem unconstructive or counterproductive, you may want to look elsewhere for a different program or concentrate on other ways to teach social skills, outlined later in this chapter.

There are a few published manuals to teach social skills to high-functioning children and adolescents with ASD (such as Children's Friendship Training, included in the Resources) and a variety of approaches are also described on the Internet (also included in the Resources at the end of the book). As with interventions in the schools summarized in the last chapter, there are some basic principles for teaching social skills that capitalize on your child's strengths. We summarize these principles and give you examples of how they might be implemented in a therapy group in the box on page 207. Social skills training for children with ASD should break down the complex social behaviors that most children learn automatically into concrete steps and rules that can be memorized and practiced in a variety of settings. Abstract concepts, like friendships, thoughts, and feelings, should be introduced through visual, tangible, "hands-on" activities as much as possible. For example, the therapist might hold a cardboard arrow at the side of your child's face, pointed at the person to whom he is speaking, to help him learn and practice eye contact. Written schedules use your child's natural reading abilities to help him or her transition from one task to another while minimizing anxiety. A predictable routine will capitalize on your child's memory and rule-following strengths to help him or her anticipate the different group activities. There should be a behavioral plan that specifies individual goals for group members and a specific system for delivering rewards. Social skills training will be difficult for your child and, as with all people, he or she may need to be enticed to participate in this less-than-favored and possibly very challenging activity.

A final important ingredient is collaboration with parents to promote generalization. Weekly therapy in a clinic will do little to change basic deficits of ASD unless there is *daily* practice and reinforcement of the skills being learned in situations outside the therapy room. Thus, it is very important that you be aware of what your child is learning and that you be taught how to practice the skills or implement specific techniques at home, in the neighborhood, or at school. This may be accomplished partially through homework. It is also important that the therapists or teachers provide explicit opportunities to address the skills outside the group, in more natural settings for the child (for example, in the classroom, park, video arcade, bowling alley, or restaurant), perhaps through community outings. It is important that the teacher or

Basic Principles for Teaching Social Skills

Principle	Examples
Make the abstract concrete.	• Provide rules, such as "Make eye contact for 5 seconds when you begin a conversation." • Break complex behaviors into steps, such as "A conversation consists of a beginning, a middle, and an end," and teach each step. • Use visual cues, such as a double-tipped arrow, to depict the turn taking and back-and-forth of a conversation. • Use hands-on activities to practice, such as role-playing a conversation.
Help with transitions.	• Provide a written schedule that outlines the group activities in order. • Use a predictable routine every session, such as an opening discussion, a group activity, a role play, a snack, jokes, and good-bye.
Motivate.	• Set realistic goals for each child. • Provide rewards for attaining goals.
Generalize.	• Establish communication and collaboration between parents and therapists. • Give assignments to be completed outside the clinic, such as calling another group member and having a phone conversation. • Take outings into the community to practice skills, such as having conversations at a restaurant.

therapist working with your child tell you how and where to help your child practice away from the clinic or school. If this is not happening, request a private session with the therapist or group leader. Say that you want to be more involved in your child's therapy and request specific assignments or procedures for following up on skills at home.

A variety of topics should be covered in any social skills group for children and adolescents with ASD. Perhaps most basic is teaching the nonverbal behaviors that are important to social interaction, such as appropriate eye contact, social distance, voice volume, and facial expression. We call this *social body language*. A typical program might also include the following topics:

- Friendship skills: greeting others, joining a group, taking turns, sharing, negotiating and compromising, following group rules, understanding the qualities of a good friend.
- Conversational skills: starting, maintaining, and ending a conversation; taking turns talking; commenting; asking others questions; expressing interest in others; choosing appropriate topics.
- Understanding thoughts and feelings: showing empathy, taking others' perspectives, handling difficult emotions.
- Social problem solving and conflict management: coping with being told "no," being teased, being left out.
- Self-awareness: learning about autism spectrum disorder, personal strengths, unique differences, and self-acceptance.

Cognitive–Behavioral Therapy

Another clinic-based therapeutic model that may be useful to teach social skills to adolescents and young adults with ASD (those who are able to tolerate a bit more abstraction) is called *cognitive-behavioral therapy*. It was originally developed to help people with depression, who are often highly critical of themselves, pessimistic, and likely to interpret neutral events in a negative light (the "glass-is-half-empty" kind of person). At the crux of this therapy is showing people how their thoughts influence their feelings and how negative "self-talk" is related to (even causes) feelings of sadness and depression. The antidote, in a cognitive-behavioral therapy model, is to learn more positive self-talk, changing negative thoughts into positive ones and learning new ways of thinking about the self and the world. Cognitive-behavioral therapy turned out to be remarkably effective and is still a widely used treatment for depression, anxiety, and other psychological disorders.

Cognitive-behavioral therapy helps people focus on the causes and consequences of their behavior, as well as on the emotions and thoughts that accompany their behavior. Its relevance to people with high-functioning ASD should be readily apparent. Often, those with ASD have trouble reading the social cues in the environment accurately, resulting in odd or unexpected behavior. They often report difficulty understanding their feelings and trouble differentiating among similar emotions. For example, some people with ASD say that they can tell when they feel "bad" but are not sure if they are sad or angry, can't calibrate just how "bad" they feel (furious or mildly irritated), and, most confusingly, sometimes aren't sure why. And they often have poor understanding of the consequences of their behavior. So cognitive-behavioral approaches may be of some use for ASD.

Josh, a 15-year-old with ASD, came to group one day and announced that he had had a bad week because he got expelled from school. When queried about the circumstances, he replied simply that he had pushed another boy's head into a water fountain. No other explanation was forthcoming, and Josh seemed almost puzzled by what had happened. The cognitive-behavioral model was used to help Josh and the other group members understand the links among situations, responses, and consequences. The group leader stressed the importance of four aspects of Josh's situation: *who*, did *what*, *when*, and *where*. Josh began with a simple description: "This kid made me mad at school." With the structural aid of a

written list, he was eventually able to describe many specifics of the situation: details about the boy involved, what he
had done (he called Josh "fatso"), time of day, and exactly
where the incident had occurred. The group then explored
three aspects of Josh's response: his emotions, his actions, and
his thoughts (or self-talk). While he could readily identify his
actions (shoving the boy's head into the water fountain), his
emotions (shame, embarrassment, and anger) and especially
his self-talk were murky to him. Finally, the group discussed
both the short- and long-term consequences of Josh's response.
Josh had a clear understanding of one consequence (his expul-
sion from school), but seemed to have very limited awareness
of other outcomes of his actions (for example, that the other
boy had been injured and that Josh might be more likely to be
teased again in the future because of his extreme reaction).
Using a cognitive-behavioral model significantly improved
Josh's understanding of the situation and his ability to prevent
a recurrence in the future. The group also addressed ways to
change Josh's response, including substituting more positive
self-talk, using relaxation techniques, and alerting a teacher
when faced with teasing.

Cognitive-behavioral therapy, delivered in either a group or
an individual format, may be helpful for teens and adults with
ASD, not only because of the mood and anxiety problems that
are so common in this group, but also because of the explicit links
this therapy model makes among situations, responses, and consequences, concepts that are difficult for those with autism spectrum
disorder. Cognitive-behavioral treatment is more structured and
concrete than other forms of psychotherapy. Relying less on insight
and judgment than other treatment models, it focuses instead on
practical problem solving, making it an "autism-friendly" form of
therapy. However, cognitive-behavioral approaches are probably
too complex for most younger children with ASD, so it is best
to wait until adolescence and adulthood, when abstraction ability
matures, to try this type of treatment.

Strategies for Teaching Social Skills Outside the Clinic

Earlier we stressed the importance of addressing social issues in a group setting, since this is where social problems usually arise, and thus this is where your child needs to practice social behavior. We also emphasized that you should practice and support your child's emerging social abilities at home whenever possible and that social skills training in a clinic alone, one hour a week, would not do much good. In the following sections, we describe a variety of resources and techniques for working on social skills that can be used by anyone, across a variety of settings. These techniques will help your child improve her social behavior even when she is not within the four walls of the clinic or school, with a trained professional there to assist her. You are a key player in this endeavor. The following approaches do not require a professional degree to implement, just an interest in trying, a willingness to keep trying, flexibility, and a sense of humor. It is often helpful to initiate one intervention at a time so that you can monitor its success and get some sense of whether changes in the targeted behavior are occurring (and why). As always, it is useful to implement the intervention across settings whenever possible, to increase the rate of skill acquisition and improve the likelihood of generalization. And, should you run into any problems or need advice as you try any of these interventions at home, seek the help of an experienced ASD specialist.

Feedback and Modeling

Parents and siblings can be valuable role models for the child with ASD. To be effective, however, you need to be very explicit and concrete about the skills you are modeling and about drawing your child's attention to them. You can do this in a variety of ways, but perhaps the most powerful is to videotape interactions for later review. This not only appeals to most children, all of whom like to "star" in their own movies, but also permits "real-time" provision of pointers. It is a more effective strategy to pause a video and highlight a problem or make a suggestion right at that moment than it is to try to reconstruct the situation later. Choose your battles—decide first what skill you want to highlight (for example, eye contact, turn taking, appropriate conversational topics, or sharing during play) and then focus your comments on that specific skill. Be sure to praise your child for things he is doing well (or even doing OK) and gently provide guidance in behaviors where he could improve. Try to phrase suggestions positively, giving examples of what your child can do to improve, rather than focusing on mistakes and using a lot of "don't" statements. It can sometimes be helpful to videotape siblings or peers engaged in similar interactions. Point out things those children did well ("See how Amanda is looking right in my eyes and nodding while I talk to her?") to explicitly draw your child's attention to the way the behavior is supposed to be performed. But also point out things that did not go smoothly in the interaction, so that your child with ASD doesn't feel singled out or criticized unfairly.

Parents and siblings can provide a daily time to practice conversational skills at home, much as time is set aside for homework or piano practice. This might involve a 10-minute period each day in which you and your child talk in a structured manner. You may need to write down topics beforehand, to promote topic maintenance, avoid drifting to more preferred subjects, and help your child formulate some ideas in advance. You may want to use some visual aids, such as a cardboard arrow or spinner to indicate whose turn it is to talk or a script with suggested questions or comments. As just described, you can videotape the conversations for later review and practice.

You may have been frustrated many times by the small amount of personal information that your child shares spontaneously with you. So it may seem ironic that you may also have to watch out for oversharing of personal information. When they decide to share, many children with ASD don't know where to draw the line and end up creating an awkward situation for themselves and those around them. One young lady with high-functioning ASD, who wondered about her romantic attraction to a classmate, suddenly began to explore this attraction aloud in the lunchroom. Many of her classmates felt uncomfortable with this sudden, excessive disclosure and started to avoid her. One way to prevent this situation is through the provision of very explicit feedback to your child. Most children and teens with ASD do not catch on to subtle suggestions about behavior. Therefore, you need to be explicit in defining for your child which topics are appropriate and which are not, perhaps in the form of a list. Make sure your child learns to recognize some signs that the other person may be disinterested in or uncomfortable with what he or she is saying, such as looking surprised, trying to change the topic, or blushing, and then has a list of more appropriate conversational topics to revert to.

How to Get the Most Out of Clubs, Activities, and Play Dates

Just putting your child in situations with other children isn't enough to ensure that his social issues will be addressed. The suggestions in this section are a bit more focused than just enrolling your child in extracurricular activities that expose him to peers. Social groups, like scouts, can be helpful, but usually there must be some explicit structuring and specific interventions to make such situations beneficial. It may be more useful to choose some social group activity that revolves around your child's interests and talents, to make the experience palatable and to expose your child to others who are like-minded and therefore more inclined to accept and appreciate him. Many communities have computer, reading, or science clubs that may interest your child. If there is a university in your area, inquire about programs it may have for youth, which often revolve around similar themes.

Drama clubs can also be very helpful for children with ASD. Your child may initially be self-conscious or otherwise reluctant to try such a group, but the benefits can be substantial. After all, what is acting other than being told what to say, how to behave, how to make your voice sound, and how to make your face look in certain social situations? We have seen several children with high-functioning ASD prosper in drama groups.

If the situation is structured appropriately, parents can help guide younger children with ASD through a "play date" and make it a successful learning experience. But don't stop with inviting another child over to play. It is important to choose an activity for your child and the friend to do together; don't rely on their ability to come up with something interactive. Many children would sit side by side and play video games the whole time. Choose an activity that requires some interaction, such as playing a board game, cooking a simple recipe, or working on an art project. Build in explicit social opportunities, such as giving one child the flour and the other child the measuring cups, or having each child decorate a cookie for the other person. This gives your child the chance to practice requesting, sharing, turn taking, and perspective taking. Be sure that the activity is appealing to both participants. *And* be sure that your child knows how to perform the requisite behaviors beforehand, perhaps by playing the game or making the recipe first with you or a sibling. Don't make learning the rules of the game part of the play date; have the goals of the play date be social, pure and simple. That is, have your child take existing skills and now use them with a peer. You may need to be present during most of the interaction, prompting and reminding both children about turn taking, sharing, negotiating, and the like. You may even find it helpful to use some visual aids to structure the interaction (such as a spinner to indicate whose turn it is, a recipe with pictures showing all the ingredients, or a written list of game rules). Your goal is to reduce your intervention and monitoring until the children can play together without adult assistance. This may take some time, but is more likely to happen eventually if you first provide structure than if you simply invite a peer to your home.

Keep in mind that most children—those with typical development included—need a lot of structure to have a successful play date. Squabbles and difficulties sharing and accommodating to others are part and parcel of children's social development.

Social Scripts

Social scripts are nothing more than written prompts or guidelines for what to do and say in a common social situation. Although you may not be conscious of using them, most of us have a variety of social scripts in our repertoire that we use when faced with a specific social situation. For example, we all generally know what to do and say when we meet someone new: we might extend our hand, say hello, introduce ourselves, ask the other person's name, and so on. Most people also have a pretty consistent social script that they use when ordering food in a restaurant and when answering the telephone. People with ASD, however, usually haven't constructed such social scripts or have them accessible. Thus, it can be very helpful to provide such a script, in a format conducive to how most people with high-functioning ASD learn (using written cues or other visual structures, for example). Given their typically good memory skills, children with ASD may well be able to memorize components of the script so that the written instructions can eventually be dispensed with. Scripts are not difficult to write and require little more than putting yourself in your child's shoes and writing down the script you (or a child) would use in that situation.

Clint very much wanted to ask a woman he knew at work to a dance at his church, but he was very apprehensive about calling her on the telephone. His father reminisced about his own difficulty calling women for dates when he was a young man and suggested that Clint use a "phone script" that outlined the important things he needed to say. Clint warily agreed. His father wrote out the following script:
 "Hello, is Cindy there please?"

"Hi, Cindy, this is Clint, from work." (*Pause until you make sure she knows who you are.*) "Am I catching you at a good time to talk for a moment?"

If no: "When could I give you a call back?" (*Pause for answer.*) "OK, see you at work tomorrow. Bye."

If yes: "There's a dance at my church this Saturday evening. I was wondering if you are free and might like to go?"

If no: "Too bad. How about doing something else the weekend after? Maybe a movie?"

If yes: "Great. My dad will give us a ride. We'll pick you up at 7:00. What is your address?"

And so forth. Other examples of scripts you might provide to your child or teen include how to indicate uncertainty, ask for help, or buy something in a store. It is always best to practice the scripts several times with your child before expecting her to use them in public. Videotaping and reviewing the scripted interaction can again be extremely helpful.

Social Stories

Social Stories, mentioned in Chapter 6, are written, sometimes illustrated, stories that present information about social situations. They were developed by Carol Gray, an educational consultant in the Michigan public school system (see the Resources for more information). They are different from social scripts in being much less directive. Instead of just telling what to do and say, they supply critical information about the social situation, highlighting certain social cues and other people's motives or expectations. Most important, Social Stories provide a rationale for why the child should do or say what he is told to do or say. Carol Gray explains the need for such justification through the following example. If someone told us to go stand on our head in the corner, either we would refuse or we'd do it once (while the other person prompted and watched us) and then never again. Why? Because that behavior made no sense in that particular situation. It is much the same with our children with ASD—we may tell them to do or say something that seems completely alien to them. So it is incumbent upon us to provide the *reason* behind certain social behaviors if we want our children to use them regularly. In fact, Ms. Gray suggests (and many researchers also believe) that this failure to understand the *"why"* of social behavior is at the crux of many of the difficulties associated with the ASD.

Ms. Gray outlines some very specific rules for writing an effective Social Story. For example, it should contain more informative statements (explaining social cues or providing reasons) than directive statements (telling the child what to do and say). Directives should be stated positively ("Do this" rather than "Don't do that"). It is outside the scope of this chapter to outline all the specific instructions for writing Social Stories; we refer you to the Resources for additional information if you are interested in these stories, which are widely used by parents in homes and are not difficult to design. Here is one example of a Social Story written to help a child learn appropriate behavior in the cafeteria at school.

Tracy, who has high-functioning ASD and is 9 years old, had trouble with many aspects of the lunch situation. She didn't like to wait in line, she wanted to eat only desserts, and she cried and threw a tantrum when a hole was punched in her lunch card. The Social Story her parents wrote helped her understand *why* she needed to do these things. It also gave her some clear concrete rules she could follow. Her teachers put each bulleted item from the Social Story on a separate piece of paper, let Tracy draw a picture to illustrate each page, and allowed her to carry it on her tray at lunch. This intervention was very helpful in changing Tracy's cafeteria behavior, and her tantrums reduced dramatically almost immediately. Tracy's parents began making Social Stories to help her understand how to behave in many other difficult social situations, including being nice to her new baby brother, taking a shower, following mealtime routines, sitting still in synagogue, and riding an escalator at the mall.

Eating in the School Cafeteria

- When it's time for lunch, my teacher tells the class that it is time to go to the cafeteria.
- I walk to the cafeteria with all the other kids. I try to walk slowly.
- We have to wait in line for our food. I wait my turn to get my lunch. It is important to wait my turn. Other kids don't like me if I push ahead of them. I want other kids to like me.
- The lady behind the counter is very nice. She asks me what I want. I get to choose a main course, a vegetable, a dessert, and a drink. I point to each food, and she puts it on my tray.
- I can have only one dessert. If I have too much dessert, I might feel sick.
- I say "thank you" to the lunch lady.
- I push my tray to the end of the line and give my lunch card to the person at the cash register. She punches a hole in it. This hole tells them that I paid for my lunch.
- I take my tray to my table and eat with Susan and Jane.

Social Stories are thought to be helpful not only in providing justifications for social behavior, but also in being highly visually structured. They provide a written product that the child can refer back to at any time to remind him of appropriate social behaviors in the classroom (raising hand, waiting in line, handling a change in class schedule, and so on). Social Stories can be written on index cards and taped to a child's desk, and many children keep their Social Stories organized in a notebook or on a tablet computer and enjoy rereading them with family or saving ones they no longer need as evidence of the progress they are making.

Narrating Life

The goal of Social Stories is to explain social cues and justify the importance of certain social behaviors to your child. There are other ways to accomplish this goal. One is a technique called "narrating life," developed by Linda Andron, a social worker at UCLA who specializes in helping individuals with ASD. Dr. Brenda Smith Myles, a professor at the University of Kansas Medical Center, calls this approach "thinking out loud." As these names for the technique indicate, it involves providing a running commentary of your behavior and thought processes. For example, you can verbally describe what you are doing, why you are doing it, how you are making decisions, why you are selecting certain behaviors instead of others, and what cues you are noticing. This technique is quite a bit like a Social Story, but it is not visual, nor does it have a concrete product. This may mean that it will be less useful for some children, but its appeal is that it is incredibly simple to implement and can be used anywhere, at any time.

When Seth's mother went to the grocery store, she talked aloud to him as she performed every step of the process. As she chose a brand of soup, she said, "I think I'll buy this brand today. We've been having the other brand for so long that I think we're getting tired of it. Plus, this one is on sale." As she looked for a special item, she said aloud, "When I can't find something, I ask someone who works here. You can usually tell who is a store employee by their nametag." As Seth's mother chose which checkout line to stand in, she said, "This cashier looks fast and her line is pretty short. And she is smiling at everyone, so she looks friendly." As they waited in line, she said to Seth, "Sometimes it's hard to wait in such a long line. But it would be rude to push ahead, and others would get mad at me. And waiting gives me a chance to look at the magazines next to the checkout." As she opened her purse, she said, "Before we leave, I need to pay for all these things. If I don't have enough cash, I can use a check or a credit card." As they left the store together, his mother said to Seth, "That cashier sure was nice. I always like chatting with the cashier. If I can't think of anything to say, I mention the weather."

Friendship Files

Tony Attwood, author of *The Complete Guide to Asperger's Syndrome*, suggests that parents help their child create index cards that contain relevant information about peers. Keeping information about other kids' attributes, interests, and favorite activities in this format can make information easier to recall for your child and enable her to prepare in more concrete ways for interactions. Help your child use the cards to:

- Choose appropriate topics of conversation.
- Compliment others (through knowledge of their attributes).
- Choose activities that the peer might enjoy.

Friendship files thus not only promote friendship but, more broadly, teach your child important perspective-taking skills, such as being attuned to the interests of others and tailoring interactions around the partner.

Peer Coaching

A very different type of strategy that can be used to teach social skills is what we call *peer mediation*. What that means is that "typical" children (those without ASD) of the same age interact in a more natural setting with children or teens who have ASD. Just placing them in proximity to each other won't be enough (this is probably already happening at school, and yet your child is still having social difficulties). Instead, the typical peers are explicitly taught how to initiate interactions, prompt social responses, give feedback, and reinforce children with ASD. They are given several simple guidelines for interacting with the person with ASD, such as staying near them, joining their activity, making comments, praising them for even small interactive behaviors, and being persistent. General information about ASD may be shared with the typical peers. Possible situations (for example, the child with ASD ignores the peer or talks on and on about reptiles) are role-played to give the typical peers some ideas about how to interact. After this, however, the adult does not serve as a therapist or interact directly with the children with ASD, but instead lets the peers behave and interact with them. The therapists remain present to support, encourage, and protect the child with ASD when necessary but try to deliver the treatment through the typical peers, effectively eliminating themselves as the "middle man." Often peer-mediated interventions are done in schools, but they can also be implemented in a clinic or community setting—they have even been adapted for use in the home (see below).

Research demonstrates that peer mediation approaches have clear benefits. One study showed that the rate of asking for things, getting another child's attention, waiting for a turn, and making eye contact increased two- to threefold after a peer intervention in a kindergarten classroom. It also appears that children with ASD generalize new skills to other settings and maintain them well over time, probably because the need to transfer newly learned social skills from an adult therapist to same-age typical peers is eliminated.

You may want to approach your child's school to see if it would be willing to implement some type of peer-mediated intervention in the classroom. Or you may want to adapt this approach for use in your home, with siblings or neighborhood children serving in the role of the peer coach. If you do so, be sure to prepare and train the "peer" in advance. You know your child's particular quirks and social difficulties, so prepare the peer for problems that might arise and role-play how to deal with them. Give the peer a few rules to guide the interaction (for example, stay near John, keep trying to play with him, and ignore it when he talks to himself). Initially, monitor the interactions, much as described above in the section on structured play dates. Then step back and let the children interact.

Circle of Friends

This is an activity intended to help children who have few friends become part of a group and be included in social activities. It is best implemented in a classroom or other natural group setting (for example, scout camp or religious classes). A social "map" made of concentric circles is constructed, with the child at the center, the inner ring containing family, the next ring containing other supports (teachers, therapists, clergy), and the outer ring friends. In a classroom, a teacher might first construct a Circle of Friends for a few typical children. Then she constructs one for the child with ASD. It becomes immediately apparent that the outer ring is visibly less dense relative to the typical peers, perhaps even empty. The teacher then asks for volunteers to be in the Circle of Friends of the child with ASD. These volunteers are given a variety of assignments, from greeting the child when she enters the class, to engaging her in play or conversation on the playground, to sitting with her at lunch. The success of the Circle of Friends program appears to revolve around close monitoring of the "volunteer friends." Pretraining (much as is done with peer mediators in social skills groups, described above) is necessary. It should cover basics about ASD, tips to engage the child, advice about what to do when unusual behaviors occur, and some role playing of potential situations. Once the intervention starts, short but regular (weekly) meetings are needed. The classroom or resource teacher or another school staff member should meet with the volunteers, listen to how they helped the child with ASD that week, discuss problems that arose, and perhaps even role-play or otherwise give suggestions for how to deal with the problems.

A similar intervention could be done at home, with neighborhood peers serving as volunteer friends. Working closely with the peers, giving them appropriate guidance and follow-up, is just as important if the Circle of Friends is constructed at home as it is at school. Be sure that the children you choose to become your child's friends are willing, eager, and well armed with information about your child so that they can be successful.

Linda, Joseph's mother, decided to organize a Circle of Friends for him in their close-knit neighborhood. She contacted three of her neighbors who had children roughly the same age as Joseph, told them about the program, and asked them to ask their children if they would be willing to play. Two 8-year-old boys agreed to be in Joseph's Circle of Friends. They already knew Joseph around the neighborhood and therefore were aware of some of his quirks, but Linda decided to tell them more specifics about ASD. She stressed that Joseph was very bright and told them of all his natural talents and special skills. She also told them that he sometimes had trouble knowing what to talk about and knowing when to stop talking. She role-played with the boys what to do when either of these situations arose. For example, when Joseph started talking about geography, she prompted the peers to say, "Oh, that's pretty interesting. Did you happen to see the basketball game last night?" When Joseph started rambling, she taught the peers to hold up an index finger and say, "Whoa! Can I say something?" and then redirect the conversation in an appropriate way. She then gave each boy specific assignments, such as sitting with Joseph on the bus, riding bikes with him in the neighborhood cul-de-sac, and calling him on the phone. Linda checked in with the boys and their mothers by phone every week to see how things were going, if they had had any problems getting along, or had encountered situations that they didn't know how to handle. Linda hoped that the boys would genuinely grow to enjoy Joseph's company, but she decided that providing them with occasional treats, such as gift certificates to the video store and outings to the pizza parlor and video arcade, would help them remain committed to playing with Joseph. This was a lot of work for Linda, but the pleasure on Joseph's face when he got a phone call or was asked to come ride bikes was worth it.

Strategies to Improve Your Child's Ability to Handle Emotion

One of the primary tasks of childhood is to learn to regulate emotional responses. For many children with ASD, the process of emotional self-regulation is delayed, and they are likely to need extra help learning to deal with strong emotions appropriately. For example, while most toddlers and many preschoolers regularly have tantrums when they are frustrated or don't get their way, by the time they enter elementary school most typically developing children have few or no tantrums. Older children and even adolescents with high-functioning ASD, on the other hand, may continue to have tantrums because they have not yet learned how to regulate their emotions. Obviously, this kind of behavior does not help them fit in socially and can be one of the causes of social rejection and isolation.

One important aspect of emotion regulation is being aware of your body's internal states and the cues indicative of emotional arousal. For example, when a person becomes frustrated, his muscles may tense up. He may feel a hot rush of blood to his face and a sudden surge of energy. Being aware of and interpreting these physiological effects of emotional arousal is difficult for many children with autism spectrum disorder.

Mateo's brothers loved going to the neighborhood arcade and often pestered their mother to take them there. She felt torn because Mateo, a young boy with high-functioning ASD, had such a hard time at the arcade. He enjoyed the experience at first, but he became so caught up in the flashing lights and sounds that he soon was out of control. He would giggle uncontrollably, run around wildly, and tackle other children. The outing inevitably ended in tears and felt like a disaster to all involved. Mateo's brothers pleaded with their mother to leave Mateo at home next time.

Tim, an adolescent with ASD, was a gifted student. Despite the fact that his arithmetic scores far surpassed his grade level, he had received several failing grades. His frustration threshold was so low that he frequently snapped in class when his pencil needed sharpening or he could not get the teacher's help quickly. He seemed unable to monitor the increasing tension in his body until it overtook him in a physical outburst, at which point he would throw his books and papers to the floor, scream "I've had it!," and march out of the classroom. The other students stared, whispered, and began to snicker.

In both of these examples, we see children who fail to monitor their level of arousal and encounter social difficulties as a result. There are a few strategies parents can use to help children learn to regulate their emotions better. First, you can encourage your child to use words to express her feelings. It is precisely when preschoolers learn to verbalize that their tantrums precipitously decrease. Begin by teaching your child to notice when she is experiencing an emotion, such as joy, anger, or sadness. Then verbally label these emotional states for your child and encourage your child to express these feelings in words (for example, "I am feeling angry!"). If your child needs it, you can also provide visual cues, such as a sheet of paper with several emotions depicted on it, to help your child figure out her emotional state (see the "Software and Applications" section of the Resources for further ideas).

After your child has expressed his feelings in words or by using pictures, provide some ways of coping with the emotionally arousing situations. At first you can make suggestions, even perhaps a list of coping strategies. For example, you can say, "If you are frustrated, you can ask for help or ask for a break or go on to a new problem." Eventually, however, you will want to ask your child to come up with solutions by himself. Prompt your child to think of further alternatives to the strategies you have provided ("What *else* could you do if you get frustrated?").

Sometimes, however, your child's emotional state will be so strong that she'll need techniques to calm herself before she can discuss her feelings and ways to cope with them. One technique that is often helpful is called *progressive relaxation*. While your child reclines and breathes deeply, verbally walk her through tensing (while breathing in) and relaxing (while exhaling) muscle groups from toe to head. As she becomes more comfortable with the process, you can teach your child to tense and relax the entire body quickly and subtly for use in stressful circumstances. An added benefit of this rapid relaxation technique is that the teaching process helps children better recognize the body states associated with tension and relaxation. A second calming strategy for your child is to engage in a relaxing activity, such as listening to music on an mp3 player or smartphone, chewing gum, drawing, having a back rub, or thinking of something comforting, such as a soft blanket or the fur of a favorite pet. A less direct strategy is to teach your child to ask for help or to remove herself from the situation when she becomes aware of potential overarousal. Tim, described above, might benefit from having a teacher's permission to leave the room for 2 minutes if he is experiencing frustration. Parents and teachers can facilitate this system by providing clear places and plans for children to take a breather and specific signals or "break cards" to let others know they need time alone. Just knowing that this option is available may be helpful for your child with ASD. Most children will benefit from using a combination of these strategies for learning and maintaining emotional control.

Dealing with Teasing and Bullying

Many children and teens with ASD are teased, belittled, or bullied in school. A recent study by Dr. Paul Shattuck and colleagues found that almost half of children with ASD have been victimized by bullies. The peer mediation approaches described above appear to foster greater peer acceptance, which may reduce the frequency of victimization by peers that can be a common part of the life of a child with ASD. Peer buddies are especially useful to the child with ASD during unstructured times of the school day, such as lunch or recess. It is well established that bullies rarely target a child who is part of a group (or even just in a pair); they tend to go after children who are alone and thus vulnerable.

There are several other techniques that have shown promise in reducing the likelihood that teasing or bullying will occur. Many approaches involve similar ingredients to those used in peer mediation programs, including providing information about autism to classmates and creating regular opportunities for interaction between children with ASD and typical peers. Other programs involve assertiveness training and teaching the child specific techniques for standing up to bullies: asking for help, seeking out a safe teacher or place, walking away, using humor, and the like. If you have reason to suspect that your child is being bullied, contact your child's teacher and principal immediately. It is of the utmost importance that your child be protected, which means outlining specific plans to deal with different situations, establishing "safe" zones around the school, and better monitoring less-structured activities and situations where the harassment may take place. The Resources at the end of this book include a variety of programs that schools and parents can use to stop bullying and create a safe environment for all children. Many schools are already implementing such programs due to the recent rash of school violence (few of which involved students with ASD, but many of which did involve children who were being bullied or teased).

The typical bullied child is insecure, anxious, and socially "adrift," with few friends or other supports. Children may also be teased because there is something different about them. This may well be the case with your child. In addition to the school-based solutions described above, you can help make your child more resistant to bullying by creating pride in the way he or she is different. A confident child is a difficult child to tease. Brent, a 10-year-old with ASD, was being taunted on the playground and called "virus boy" (due to his interest in viruses and bacteria). As his teacher later told it, Brent turned around and said, "Well, I like viruses because I have ASD and because I have ASD, I am much better at reading and video games than you." Brent, incidentally, had been enrolled in a social skills group that had emphasized these special strengths of ASD. The bully was left speechless and walked away.

If unusual behaviors such as hand flapping, talking to himself, or making noises appear to be the primary cause of your child's being teased, you might also try to help him or her become more aware of these behaviors and minimize their occurrence in public or when around peers. You might videotape your child and then point out instances of the behavior, teaching your child to identify the behavior reliably. As your child becomes aware of the behavior, you can institute a reward system (much like the self-management program described in Chapter 4) to decrease its occurrence. If the unusual behavior seems to serve a specific function, such as expressing excitement or alleviating boredom, more appropriate substitute behaviors can be taught—clapping instead of flapping or saying "Oh, yeah!" instead of making unusual noises—as discussed in Chapter 6.

Another way to help your child become aware of his or her differences, especially those that might lead to being teased, is through an explicit discussion about your child's diagnosis. As parents, you can talk with your child about the basic features of ASD, emphasizing whenever possible their special strengths and uniquely positive aspects. This can lead to a discussion of the unusual behaviors associated with ASD and how they can put your child or teen at risk for teasing. A helpful metaphor in talking about ways people can stand out is that of gorillas and flamingos. "Gorillas" stand out because they display some highly noticeable negative behavior such as aggression and tantrums, while "flamingos" stand out because they are unique and interesting but different from others. To the extent that your child does not want to stand out, you can help him identify and learn to monitor the behaviors that make him like a gorilla or (more often) a flamingo, using the techniques just described. You and your child may also want to read personal accounts written by people with high-functioning ASD (such as Temple Grandin's books) or watch movies featuring characters with ASD, to make the characteristics of the condition more tangible and easier for your child to identify. There are also two books that may be helpful in introducing your child to his ASD: *I Am Special*, by Peter Vermeulen, and *Asperger's: What Does It Mean to Me?*, by Catherine Faherty (see the Resources section for more information). We discuss issues of self-esteem and self-identity further in the next chapter, which deals with issues specific to adolescents and adults.

9

Looking Ahead

HIGH-FUNCTIONING AUTISM SPECTRUM DISORDER IN LATE ADOLESCENCE AND ADULTHOOD

> I have braved raging winds.
> I have survived the strongest storms.
> I blew through the valley of paradise.
> I have been soaking wet.
> I have survived.
> I am who I am!
> —An adolescent with ASD

Growing up presents many new challenges for children with ASD and their parents. Junior high and high school bring a more complex and less structured educational environment, requiring the child with ASD to make frequent transitions, such as moving from class to class, and to develop greater independence and flexibility. The difficulties that children with ASD have with organization and other executive function skills (discussed in Chapter 7) can make it especially challenging for them to achieve full independence. Social demands increase with age too. In early adolescence the desire to conform to social norms peaks, and this can be particularly hard for a child who is inherently different from his or her peers. This may be the first time, in fact, that many children with ASD become aware of how different they are from other children. On top of all these new demands, teenagers are expected to behave more maturely and to take on increasingly complex social and emotional roles in relationships.

The Good News about Growing Older

Fortunately, adolescence and young adulthood have a positive side too. By this time, some people with ASD, especially those who have received appropriate treatment for several years, have a solid set of tools for navigating social situations. Greater familiarity with the "rules" of social interaction can help them fit in and draw less negative attention from their peers than during childhood. At the same time, the typically developing adolescents and young adults around them are maturing and developing greater acceptance of differences in others. You can't count on tolerance, of course; cruelty among teenagers is widespread and well publicized. As a parent, you will want to continue to deal with any teasing and bullying in the ways suggested in Chapter 8. But, in general, these sorts of problems do decrease in high school and drop to very low levels in adulthood.

There are no guarantees that this will work for your son or daughter, but eccentricities and idiosyncrasies can sometimes be a social asset in high school. Take Charles, for example. In grade school, his tendency to question authority and challenge the logic of rules frequently landed him in the principal's office. His constant disruptions of class to argue about a seemingly arbitrary rule or assignment annoyed his classmates and made him unpopular. But when Charles got to high school, he was suddenly surrounded by others who felt it was their duty to point out to authority figures the errors in their logic and the injustice in their expectations concerning students. Charles was still viewed as odd by his peers, but he was also somewhat admired as the class maverick.

Another advantage of maturity is that in adulthood it becomes more acceptable to arrange one's social life around certain interests. Many typical adults socialize largely with coworkers, for example, and conversation often centers on office happenings or the subject of the work that they all have in common. For people with ASD who have chosen occupations dealing with their particular interest, this means less talk about unfamiliar or uninteresting topics and potentially less social anxiety or discomfort. Because adults have limited leisure time, it's also very common for them to seek out people with similar interests, whether through clubs, over the Internet, or via other avenues. This, too, can help people with ASD maintain a social life that is more rewarding than daunting. For example, as a child, Ellie's interest in the Civil War was considered odd by her peers. However, as an adult, she had an active and successful social circle among individuals who enjoyed reenactments of historical battles as much as she did. Indeed, she was well respected for the breadth and depth of her knowledge on the topic.

Perhaps the most important advantage of maturity in adolescents with ASD (as well as many typical teenagers) is that increased autonomy brings a greater opportunity to shape their own experience and seek a "niche" in the world that is more compatible with their own strengths and interests. Robin, a young woman with ASD, was frustrated throughout childhood by others' lack of appreciation of her interest in photography. Her parents and teachers would continually try to get her to set aside this fascination to do schoolwork, and kids were always trying to escape her long speeches on photographic techniques. But in high school Robin gained both social stature and self-esteem when she joined the yearbook staff and found everyone hounding her for a chance to occupy some space in her viewfinder. Robin's family wisely capitalized upon this interest, helping her eventually find employment as a photographer's assistant.

Because maturity brings the freedom to choose your own level and type of socialization, teens and adults with ASD also have a wider range of social options than they did as children. Some—especially those who have had some social success and learned to find interpersonal interaction rewarding in itself—choose to socially "mainstream" themselves and stick with the path of "typical" socialization. For others, social activities still feel more uncomfortable than rewarding, and these young men and women may continue to favor solitary activities. If, after years of coaching in social skills, your child chooses a solitary path in adolescence, you may feel as if you've failed. Or you may worry that the happy adult life that was your ultimate goal for your child may never be reached. In that case, try to remember that whatever level of socialization your child is most comfortable with is the one most likely to make him happy. As a parent your job is to help provide your child with the skills to socialize, but ultimately it is his decision how to use these skills. This is true for individuals both on and off the autism spectrum. All parents face the challenge of balancing what is best in their own eyes with the personal preferences of their child. Most parents hope their child will lead a happy and productive life. It's important to remember that your definition of a happy and productive life may not agree with your child's, particularly in terms of the amount and type of social contact.

Lauren, whom we first discussed in Chapter 1, had very little desire to socialize in high school. Her mother was terribly disappointed when she declined a classmate's invitation to the prom. But when Lauren entered college, she met a "soulmate," another loner who was also majoring in physics and who shared her love of movies. She and this young man spent many weekend evenings together in the movie theater. When her mother asked what she and her friend talked about together, Lauren said, "Nothing." When her mother asked if they had ever gone out for dinner before the movie or if she had ever asked her friend in for a cup of coffee, she answered, "No." Lauren's mother tried to give her scripts and other support to take the relationship to another level. But over time it became clear that Lauren derived a great deal of satisfaction and pleasure from the relationship *as it was.* Her mother eventually could see, somewhat wistfully, that even though Lauren and her friend did not have a typical adult romantic relationship, she was content and far more social than she had ever been.

Another bit of good news about adolescence is that it may well be easier for your child with ASD than you fear—and it may even be easier than it is for a typically developing child. Many individuals with ASD are so comfortable with adults and so agreeable to rules that there is little of the rule breaking, limit testing, dangerous behavior, and questioning of authority that are so much a part of typical adolescence. We aren't saying that there won't be challenges, but it is fairly rare for the parents of teens with ASD to have to face green hair, body piercings, and drug use.

Critical Issues during Adolescence and Adulthood

Teenagers and adults with high-functioning ASD face many of the same challenges that they confronted in childhood. For parents, this means that the ideas you've been using to help your son or daughter will still help. Many, perhaps even most, people with ASD continue to need support later in life, although the amount needed may well diminish over time. As you did when your child was younger, you should continue to play to his or her strengths whenever possible, capitalizing on excellent memory or visualization skills to make it easier for your maturing child to navigate higher education and the workplace. Most of the accommodations we recommended in Chapter 7 will continue to help in high school and college. Many of the strategies we offered in Chapter 6 to make home life easier will benefit your teen or adult child when she lives in a different residential setting. Most of the suggestions for easing social awkwardness and making friendships discussed in Chapter 8 will still apply.

But, you may say, my child has just gone through a huge hormonal shift. She now has a job. The rest of the world's expectations are higher now that she is older. Can we really go on as if nothing has changed? In fact, some things do change for people with high-functioning ASD as they mature. You'll need to emphasize independence and functionality more than ever. You have to learn how to negotiate a new set of situations and settings so you can help your child do so. It becomes a bit harder to strike a balance between providing support and letting your teen or adult child struggle to figure things out for herself. In this chapter, we'll help you understand when the changes you see in your child and the new struggles you encounter require a new approach.

As any parent of a teenager knows, adolescence is a challenging time. Naturally it is complicated by ASD. In the following discussion we'll tell you how you can take your child's disorder into account in handling various adolescent social issues. Just as important, however, we'll try to help you see when it's ASD that is causing your child to behave the way he is behaving and when it's adolescence itself.

You'll see in this chapter that we believe your child will still need a good deal of support and structure. If this seems discouraging, please understand that much of what we know about adolescents and adults with high-functioning ASD comes from the study of individuals who were diagnosed as teens or adults. These people have not had the benefit of the early and prolonged treatment that your child has probably had, and so naturally they require more structure and intervention than your child might, *if* she is quite high functioning and has had many years of intervention. Now that high-functioning forms of ASD have been being diagnosed for several decades, the field is developing an increasingly clear picture of what adults with ASD who have had early intervention truly need. For now, however, you will need to sort through the following recommendations to figure out which are necessary for your teen or adult child.

Support People

As your child has grown, you (possibly with help from teachers and therapists) have served as facilitator, translator, and guide in a world that has often been difficult for him. You have been an advocate, doing whatever it takes to ensure that your child is provided with the services he needs. You've reinterpreted hundreds of misperceived social slights and smoothed over many inadvertent social faux pas. You have been a person to hug after a rough day at school and to extend a hand to high-five after a successful social event. Despite your incredible efforts and successes, with growing maturity your child needs to find support elsewhere. The more independent your son or daughter becomes, the less likely you will be there to assist.

Sometimes parents feel that they should take a less intrusive role in the life of their child as she gets older. What seemed acceptable to help with at age 10 can seem infantile for a teenager. For example, perhaps you've walked your child to school every morning but begin to wonder if that is still appropriate when she enters high school. Some adolescents with ASD will continue to want this kind of support. Let your child's individual needs and wishes dictate your behavior.

But some teens with ASD begin to demand independence from their parents and view the support that they see as "interference." Although it is likely that you will begin to see this natural need to develop independence in your child, this need will likely emerge a bit later than for typically developing teenagers. But if your teen with high-functioning ASD does begin to begrudge the support you are providing, you will have to figure out how to respond. Your teenager or young adult will likely still need advice, moral support, sympathy in times of difficulty, and shared joy after victories. How can you continue to provide the structure that you believe your adolescent needs, but in a way that will be accepted and that is constructive?

One way that you can appropriately alter your support role as your child grows older is to recruit "helpers" in the community or the natural settings your child is encountering. Support may be provided by a friend, a case manager, a therapist, a coworker, or different people in different settings. Now, while your child is just entering adolescence, is the time to help your child understand the need to actively recruit people to turn to in times of trouble. Your child might end up needing continuing professional support, such as a job coach, but even if he does not, having support people in multiple environments will alleviate much of his anxiety.

John's mother was delighted that her son was joining the high school swim team. However, she also knew that locker rooms and team bus rides would present a host of confusing social situations for her son to decipher. She mentioned to John that she thought it would be a good idea for him to have a "go-to" person in case he became confused or uncertain in that setting. He liked the assistant coach and felt comfortable talking with him, so they agreed he was a viable mentor. Together they wrote a note describing how they would like him to be available for assistance. John showed it to him after practice the next week. The coach readily agreed. John found that over the course of the season his "mentor" was invaluable, helping him understand that hugging other teammates was appropriate only at certain times, that pointing out team fouls to the referee was unnecessary, and that several of the more colorful locker room quotes were better left unrepeated in the following day's recounting of the game.

John's mother's use of the term "go-to person" was quite intentional. When you discuss the need to identify support people ahead of time, it's important to respect your son or daughter's need for independence and self-reliance, as these are critical aspects of identity for any adolescent. Instead of using terms like "helper," employ "mentor" or "coach" to stress your child's expertise rather than to imply an absence of skill. Brainstorm with your child the many different situations where an "expert opinion" might be helpful, such as at school, in a job, or in an after-school club. Pick a person that your child would feel comfortable seeking advice from in each setting. To make things more official and to be certain that the support person is willing to accept this role, explain to the candidate that you would like him or her to be the person your child can approach with any questions or confusion in that setting, as John and his mother did. One young adult with ASD worked out a similar arrangement with a supervisor at his place of employment. Whenever things got a little confusing and he wasn't quite sure how to handle them, he knew this person would be ready and willing to respond to his queries. In fact, this "go-to" person turned out to be so indispensable that a backup was selected in case the supervisor was unavailable.

Disclosure

If your child's symptoms lessen with age, as often happens, and if she branches out into new settings, the question of disclosure of your child's disorder will come up more and more often. At first you'll participate in the decision of whether or not to tell others that your child has ASD. For example, it will be your call to determine whether or not to let the camp counselor, sports coach, or neighborhood parents know that your son or daughter has ASD. Eventually, however, the decisions will be your child's to make, so introducing the issue and the decision-making process with her in early adolescence is good preparation. Your child will need to decide whether or not to disclose the diagnosis to employers and coworkers, friends and acquaintances, and perhaps even romantic interests in the future.

The pros and cons of disclosing will vary by context and circumstances, but you and your child should be aware that there are many benefits to sharing a diagnosis of ASD and relevant information with people with whom your child will have contact. In many situations, like school, organized groups or sports teams, and work settings, disclosing the challenges of ASD can help your child gain understanding from others or lead to special accommodations. It can head off misunderstandings about any unusual behaviors or perceived aloofness. It can even relieve the person of worry about having to conceal symptoms or about being on the fringes of the group.

Marcus paced across the foyer in his parents' home. Yesterday had been his first day at a new job at a computer company. For the first time, Marcus was working independently, without a job coach. Marcus is 22 years old and has high-functioning ASD. He was worried that his behavior had come across as odd to some of his coworkers while he was being given a tour of the office. His mother noticed his anxious behavior and asked him what he was worrying about. When he explained the situation, his mother offered to hold a meeting in which she would explain his diagnosis to his coworkers. Marcus was initially resistant. He had worked so hard over so many years to overcome his diagnosis. His mother had an idea that was more acceptable to him. They worked out a short script that Marcus could use when he met a new coworker or was worried about an interaction. The script went like this: "I have a disorder called autism spectrum disorder. Sometimes I'm not sure what to say or do in conversations and social interactions. I apologize if my behavior seemed rude. If you'd like to learn more about autism spectrum disorder, I'd be glad to discuss it with you." Marcus had a great memory and had little difficulty memorizing the script. In the future, Marcus wound up using this approach to disclose his diagnosis to several of his coworkers. He was pleased to discover that they were open and accepting of this information and were eager to learn more and assist him in any way possible.

Despite Marcus's positive experience, there can be some risk inherent in disclosing as well. Disclosure may invite prejudice among those who inappropriately view people with ASD as incapable of relating to others and making a meaningful contribution. As public awareness and understanding of high-functioning ASD has increased in the last three decades, this is becoming much less likely. There is even a chance, if your child's symptoms are subtle, that others may think he is making excuses for inappropriate behavior. But, in a broad sense, disclosing information about your child's diagnosis helps everyone with ASD by normalizing the phenomenon and helping others appreciate how common the disorder is and how capable those with it can prove to be. One rule of thumb we suggest is that if your child's differences would be obvious to others anyway, then providing an explanation for them by disclosing the diagnosis may well outweigh any perceived risks, such as stigma. On the other hand, if your child's symptoms have become so mild as to be mere "quirks" or personality traits that do not impair functioning, then disclosing the diagnosis might not be beneficial. Liane Willey, an adult with Asperger syndrome, has made the decision about disclosure many times and has included a number of important factors to consider in her book, *Pretending to Be Normal*, that you may also wish to access (see the Resources for more information about this book). Stephen Shore, another individual with high-functioning ASD and advocate, published a collection of passages regarding experiences with disclosure titled *Ask and Tell: Self-Advocacy and Disclosure for People on the Autism Spectrum*. Also be aware that if there are substantial negative effects of disclosing the diagnosis in a work or educational setting, you may also wish to investigate your child's legal rights under antidiscrimination laws.

Once a decision has been made to share information about your teenage or adult child's diagnosis with others, together you must decide on an appropriate strategy to convey this information. This will no doubt vary according to who is being informed. For some individuals, like Marcus, a well-rehearsed speech is an appropriate first pass at disclosure. For others, it can be helpful to provide your child with cards, much like "business cards," that explain what ASD is. These cards can be carried in a wallet, pocket, or purse and handed to another person in an awkward situation. For example, the card might state, "I have Autism Spectrum Disorder.

This is a disorder that affects my sense of social understanding, and sometimes I am uncertain how to behave or speak in social situations. Thank you for your understanding."

It is likely that many people, particularly those who will continue to have close contact with your child, will be interested in learning more about ASD. You might provide these people with some literature about ASD or some first-person published accounts, such as *Pretending to Be Normal* or *Look Me in the Eye* (see the Resources at the end of the book). Another option, if the person is interested in devoting some time to gain a deeper understanding, would be to take the person to an ASD meeting or conference. For individuals who wish to disclose openly and help others feel comfortable asking about ASD, you might display relevant materials, such as books about ASD, in a prominent place in your home. This opens the door for discussion but leaves whether to broach the subject to the visitor's discretion.

A more personal way to teach others about ASD is to describe what it means in your own terms and share what the experience has been like in your family's particular case. This information can be conveyed via a medium comfortable for you or your child, such as a story, a poem, or a conversation. For most families with a child with ASD, the decision to share additional information is a sensitive one. They would like to help others understand, but they are fearful of imposing or appearing pushy. We recommend making it clear to people that you have information and other opportunities for them to learn more about ASD without making them feel obligated to learn about the diagnosis.

> *A disclosure card—or rehearsed script—can help your young adult with ASD reveal the disorder:*
>
> "I have ASD. This is a disability that affects my sense of social understanding, and sometimes I am uncertain how to behave or speak in social situations. Thank you for your understanding."

Sexual Development

Even parents with normal children often find sexuality a difficult subject to discuss, yet it's far too important a topic to avoid. Most adolescents between 13 and 18 report frequently thinking about sex, and 50% say they engaged in sexual intercourse before age 18. Adolescents with ASD may lag in emotional or social development, but for many their biological drives develop on time. Given the reticence about personal matters so typical of those with ASD, it is even more important for you than for a parent of a child without ASD to approach your child about this topic. Sometimes parents of children with ASD wrongly assume that delays in social development and interests give them permission to delay conveying information about sexuality and puberty. We recommend, however, that you deliver this information on the same timetable as, or even earlier than, you would for children without ASD. In fact when it comes to discussing sexuality, it's not a question of *if* but of *when*. The answer, we firmly believe, is *early*. Don't put off this essential discussion until a crisis occurs. Important issues to address include sexual intercourse, birth control, nocturnal emissions, breast and testicular self-examination, masturbation, and menstruation.

Be specific and concrete in your discussions of sexual development with your child. Provide factually accurate information in a comprehensible and straightforward manner, perhaps referring to a book with illustrations. For example, set up a concrete system and schedule for hygiene related to menstruation. In addition to showing your daughter the materials she will need to use and how to use them, you might also want to furnish her with pictures or photographs showing the order in which each step is carried out. Be specific about how often she will need to change her pad or tampon. Help her use timers or alarms on her mobile device to remind her when she needs to visit the bathroom. If your daughter's menstrual cycle is regular, mark on her calendar or set monthly alerts to indicate when she will need to carry supplies with her. Write out a script that she can use in class to ask to use the restroom.

Masturbation is another important topic to discuss with your adolescent. Masturbation is a natural means of exploring developing sexuality. Teach your child very specific rules in terms of when and where masturbation or the discussion of it is appropriate. One adolescent we know was so excited when he discovered masturbation that he began telling all of his friends about his wonderful discovery. His parents certainly wished they had thought to discuss the topic with him before he brought it up. Be alert to the availability of graphic images and videos on the Internet. Most Internet browsers are equipped with parental controls to prevent visitation of pornographic websites. This is a helpful option, but it is not foolproof. Even with these safeguards in place, we recommend that you discuss with your child the kinds of information that you are comfortable with him accessing on the Internet. This may vary from family to family. One mother bookmarked artistic nude websites for her teenage son, preferring to provide him with access to these images than have him stumble upon more graphic or hard-core imagery. Though this was the right decision for this family, it might seem shockingly indiscrete to others. As with the other topics we have discussed, adhere to your own values and comfort level, but be explicit and concrete.

Since, particularly in adolescent boys, sexual arousal can be unpredictable but conspicuous, it is also helpful to work out a plan of action to help your child manage such circumstances. For example, you might tell your son that when he has an erection, he should remain seated or go to the restroom. One precaution to take when the teenage years of spontaneous erections approach is to make sure your child does not wear certain types of pants to school. Sweat pants, for example, can make sexual arousal extremely noticeable.

It's important not just to broach the subject of sexuality with your child but also to revisit it periodically to ensure that your child thoroughly comprehends the social rules surrounding sexuality. The best way to do so is to make sure that your child knows it is OK to talk with you about these matters. It may be necessary to approach a child who is not forthcoming every few months for an official update. In a worst-case scenario, misunderstandings in this area could lead to individuals with ASD becoming either unwitting sexual offenders or vulnerable to sexual victimization. If you find these topics too uncomfortable to broach, enlist the aid of a pediatrician, psychologist, or other health professional.

Romantic Relationships

Many parents have difficulty imagining a child with limited social interest eager to engage in intimate romantic relationships. People with ASD vary greatly in their level of interest in romantic relationships. For some, interest in romance and sexual relationships develops along with physical sexual development, much as for their typical peers. For others, the complex emotional aspects of romance may delay interest in intimate relationships until late adolescence or adulthood. Some of our patients have developed romantic interests and later relationships or marriages. These relationships succeed when they are mutually beneficial—the partner with ASD receives support, and the typical partner gets a companion with remarkable honesty, faithfulness, and devotion. When they don't succeed, it is usually a consequence of the difficulties that people with ASD have with emotional intimacy, intrusive interests and preoccupations, perspective taking, and compromise.

Other people with ASD never develop an interest in romantic relationships. For many, such as Temple Grandin, the option of living a productive life without a partner is more appealing and less complicated. Others may marry fellow people on the autism spectrum, and others still may find a loving relationship with someone who is typically developing or has a different challenge. As a parent of a child with ASD, your mentoring can help your child understand relevant issues and make informed choices in this area as an independent individual.

As your child develops sexual feelings, she will likely demonstrate sexual interest in others and develop a desire for intimate relationships. Recall your own experience of the anxiety that teenage romances provoked: the uncertainty, the confusion, and the bewilderment. For a child who has difficulty understanding more basic social interactions, these complexities of romance can be overwhelming. You can make this unfamiliar territory more comfortable for your child by providing concrete rules for dealing with people to whom she is attracted. Provide examples of appropriate and inappropriate behavior and how they might affect the person to whom they are directed. Your child may be highly motivated to do this exercise in perspective taking, because no one wants to make the wrong impression on the individual on whom she has a crush. Potential problem areas in which it is crucial to establish explicit guidelines include physical contact, staring, following, phone calls, visits, and types/topics of questions. Although few adolescents are adept at figuring out all the signals for returned interest or disinterest, this area may be particularly difficult for children with ASD due to their difficulty in interpreting subtle social cues. Offer your child some basic guidelines for interpreting behaviors that may indicate mutual interest or a lack of interest. This will be important in ensuring that your child's romantic leanings do not cause others discomfort.

Technology has introduced a variety of opportunities and challenges that did not exist in your youth. Mobile phones equipped with cameras and videos provide many benefits for your child but also risks for making bad decisions or being taken advantage of. Establish explicit rules regarding the content of text messages or the capture of pictures and videos. The social vulnerabilities associated with ASD can lead teens with ASD to be gullible. Make clear that, no matter how much they trust or love another, they should never take or allow others to take pictures or videos of a sexual nature. In the past, teenage foibles might have lived only in the embarrassed memory of those involved, but now a single impulsive action can live forever on the Internet.

Angelo developed his first crush when he was 14. The object of his admiration was a sweet young woman named Ella. Although she understood that he had ASD, and she liked him as a friend, she soon grew uncomfortable with his courtship. He would frequently interrupt her when she was in conversation with other people. She often felt uncomfortable because he gazed at her for long stretches of time. When she brought it to the attention of a school authority, Angelo was mortified and wanted to figure out what he was doing wrong. He and his parents drew up some guidelines to help him make sure his behavior was appropriate. They made clear that it was not appropriate to touch Ella, and they delineated situations in which it was not appropriate to approach her, such as when she was in midconversation or was reading in study hall. Looking toward the future, they made concrete rules (based on number of seconds elapsed) about what constituted staring versus casual eye contact. They also discussed some telltale signs that another person was or was not interested in one's advances. Angelo was disappointed that his relationship with Ella was not to be, but he looked forward to future romances.

Self-Awareness, Self-Esteem, and Identity Development

Adolescence may be the first time that children with ASD begin to form an identity by pondering questions like "Who am I?" and "Where do I fit in?" and "What will I become?" These aspects of adolescent development pose a significant set of challenges for young people with ASD.

One such area is definition of self-concept. Research suggests that boys and girls use different strategies to determine their own self-concept. For girls, self-concept often relates to perceptions of physical attractiveness. Young women with ASD may find this problematic due to the close link between perceived attractiveness and social mastery and popularity. Among boys, physical prowess composes an important aspect of self-concept. Again, this presents a challenge for children with ASD because of the common link between ASD and motor coordination problems (see Chapters 2 and 3).

Closely related to self-concept is self-esteem. Many adolescents experience periods of low self-esteem. Parents of children with ASD can expect the same. Sources of low self-esteem among children with ASD usually relate to wanting to be liked and to have friends but not knowing how to succeed.

Morality is another facet of adolescent identity development that is often challenging for children with ASD. Although strong moral convictions can be a notable strength for children with ASD, it can also cause some social difficulties. Superficially clear-cut moral guidelines can lead children to make poor judgments in adolescence, when interactions become more subtle and complex. Like many adolescents, children with ASD may develop strong religious or political beliefs in response to these ambiguities. After reading a book on the meat-packing industry, one young woman with high-functioning ASD decided that eating meat was unhealthy. In addition to simply changing her own diet, she attempted to influence others by pointing out to classmates and the school cafeteria staff all of the health dangers that the nonvegetarian menu items were likely to pose.

Challenges related to the development of identity and self-esteem can present difficulties for children with ASD and their families, but there are several strategies you can use to deal with these issues. As we discussed in Chapter 5 and at the end of Chapter 8, emphasizing your child's strengths and special characteristics will help him develop positive self-esteem. For example, if your child has a great memory, he can be the "Memory Master." Calling your child by this nickname when he demonstrates the skill makes clear that he has just done something special and gives him an easily referenced positive way of looking at himself.

Many teens and young adults with ASD don't realize that their feelings of awkwardness and not fitting in are common and experienced at some point by almost everyone. Few people make it to adulthood without experiencing teasing and rejection. Help your child understand that this experience is par for the course. Sharing some of your own personal experiences during your teenage years can impress on your child that everyone experiences self-doubt as a teen and relieve some of the anxiety about herself that she may be experiencing. Your child may benefit from establishing relationships with others on the autism spectrum. There are now many support groups and Internet communities for individuals with ASD. For example, the Global and Regional Asperger Syndrome Partnership (*www.grasp.org*) is an active community of self-advocates. For many people on the spectrum, it is confidence-inspiring and empowering to connect with others who have faced similar challenges. There are also published resources that were developed to assist in the exploration of self-identity: *I Am Special*, by Peter Vermeulen, and *Asperger's . . . What Does It Mean to Me?*, by Catherine Faherty (see the Resources for more information).

Depression and Anxiety

During adolescence (and sometimes earlier), many children who were previously oblivious to or even content with their lack of social connections start to experience distress. In childhood, much of friendship consists solely of acting as "playmates" and engaging in activities, such as sports or video games, together. During adolescence, however, the very nature of friendship changes in several ways that can challenge young people with ASD. Friendships become more sophisticated and complex, with an increasing emphasis on trust, mutual sharing of personal information, and common or admired personality characteristics. These changes in the nature of friendship often increase the social difficulties encountered by adolescents with ASD. These problems are compounded by the burgeoning self-awareness and the ability to make comparisons between the self and others that develop during adolescence. Feeling excluded or irreparably different can and often does lead to depression among adolescents with ASD. Real and perceived disparities with peers can lower an adolescent's sense of self-worth and promote a descent into depression. Anxiety disorders are also a common psychiatric disturbance experienced by teens and adults with ASD.

Science has not yet clarified whether these mood problems result from the natural psychological consequences of managing ASD or represent a biological disposition that is related to ASD. It may well be a combination of the stress of chronically trying to fit in, the pain of rejection, and a biological vulnerability to mood problems. Some research suggests that mood disorders run in the families of people with ASD. Depression and anxiety disorders in family members usually appear well before the birth of the child with ASD, so they do not appear to be simply a reaction to the stress of raising a special needs child. Another piece of evidence is that the neurotransmitter serotonin (a brain chemical that helps brain cells communicate with each other) appears to be altered in individuals with ASD and individuals with depression. So ASD and depression may co-occur so often for many reasons. Thus, you will need to be attentive to your child's mood and monitor whether the other interventions suggested in this book can remedy them. If not, you should consult a licensed clinical psychologist or an experienced child psychiatrist. Recent research demonstrates that directive, concrete forms of psychotherapy, such as cognitive-behavioral therapy, are effective at improving symptoms of anxiety in individuals with ASD, as described in Chapter 8. There are also highly effective medications that can help your child through difficult periods.

Seizures

Another problem sometimes encountered during adolescence in individuals with ASD is the onset of seizure disorders. Approximately 25% of all individuals with ASD experience seizures, and adolescence is a time of particular vulnerability. In some cases, seizure activity is obvious, such as when your child loses consciousness and has violent convulsions of the entire body. In other kinds of seizures, however, the signs are less obvious. Your child may have short periods (maybe only a few seconds) in which he is unresponsive (doesn't respond to his name being called or to other things going on around him). Instead, he or she may stare off into space, blink his or her eyes repeatedly, or show some kind of unusual motor behavior (such as brushing the ground with the toe of the shoe repeatedly). If you suspect your child may be experiencing seizures, he or she should be screened by a neurologist using a clinical electroencephalogram. Most seizure disorders can be effectively treated with medication.

Planning for Increasing Independence

It is critically important that you and your child begin preparing for independence well in advance. Transition planning usually focuses on the specific abilities required for functioning as a self-sufficient adult, such as daily living skills (e.g., self-care and domestic responsibilities) and employment or vocation-related skills. Individuals with ASD who have an IEP in school (see Chapter 7) are legally entitled to an Individualized Transition Plan beginning at age 14. This is mandated as part of the Individuals with Disabilities Education Act and the Americans with Disabilities Act, described in Chapter 7. The transition plan begins with an assessment, which can be formal, such as standardized testing to assess abilities and interests, or informal, such as input from family members or caregivers about the student's abilities. This planning should highlight specific targets for developing self-sufficiency, such as navigating public transportation or doing laundry. In regard to employment, it is important to consider a variety of jobs in terms of desirability, appropriateness, availability, and accessibility. Skill development goals should be planned and should be matched to jobs that are likely to be available. Goals should include both teaching marketable skills and teaching workplace behavior. Job sampling is a means for students to gain work experience. It can help your child by allowing her to practice the new skills she is learning in school in an actual work environment. This will also assist your child by providing a clearer picture of her likes and dislikes and how they are related to particular aspects of the workplace or the job itself. Throughout the process of developing an Individualized Transition Plan it will be important to include a case manager or other support person who will be involved in assisting your child after age 21, when school systems will no longer be involved.

College

The benefits of high school, from approval for concentrating on a particular interest to tolerance for—even endorsement of—eccentricity, become even greater in college. There are also, of course, some significant difficulties. During college, many young people are on their own in ways they never have been before. Your less direct supervision over your child's academic performance may mean that his difficulties will be overlooked. The following are some compensatory strategies that we have found effective. Some of these tips are based on the account of Liane Willey, a college-educated adult with Asperger syndrome and author of the book *Pretending to Be Normal.* We suggest that you review the options for educational accommodations listed in Chapter 7 as well. Many techniques that helped your child in elementary and high school will continue to be beneficial at the college level.

Disclosing

You and your child will have to consider the pros and cons of disclosing we discussed earlier, but keep in mind that many potential sources of support in the college setting open up when students share their diagnosis with professors, advisers, and tutors. These professionals may have worked with other people with ASD and can be an excellent source of guidance and support in this unfamiliar and often challenging setting. If your child feels uncomfortable disclosing, perhaps she could select one especially trustworthy person to disclose to, such as staff at the center that provides services for students with disabilities (available on all college campuses). This would ensure at least one support person on campus. Mental health professionals or others in the community might be viable alternatives if your child is hesitant to disclose to someone with direct academic connections. You can help decrease your adult child's discomfort with disclosure by normalizing the phenomenon. Let her know that there are hundreds, perhaps thousands, of other students on campus with disabilities, such as reading and attention problems. Most of these students do disclose their diagnosis to professors and make use of the services on campus for students with disabilities, which are legally mandated. For example, anyone with a recognized disability can usually take exams at the disability center, under quiet and less stressful conditions, and perhaps with extra time allowed. Many colleges now have established resources available to support students with ASD, and access to these services is likely to require disclosure of a student's diagnostic status. Some colleges have developed specific programs to help young adults with ASD acclimate to the independence and rigors of college life. In these cases, sharing this personal information with a university can make a real difference in your child's opportunity for success.

Selecting Classes

Especially at first, when your adult child is acclimating to a new environment, advise and guide him to select classes that are well suited to his strengths and to bypass areas of difficulty. When Ralph, a young man with ASD, enrolled in college, one of the first classes he took was a philosophy class. He was a concrete thinker and had a difficult time with the subtle texts assigned. At times it was unclear to him why these questions were important to consider at all. He discussed his problem with his mother and decided to orient his schedule more toward classes that focused on concrete information and memorizing a lot of information. He sold his philosophy books and experienced academic success as a chemistry major.

You may even consider requesting that certain academic requirements that are especially difficult for many people with ASD be waived. For example, foreign language study presents problems for many young adults with high-functioning ASD. Contacting the student disability center on campus is the best way to explore whether any of these requirements can be waived.

As we suggested in Chapter 7, your child may also want to enroll in small classes, where the amount of attention from the professor may be greater, or in less popular courses, where professors may be highly motivated to retain students.

Selecting Teachers

Review student evaluations and consult with other students to identify teachers who are well liked or known for their understanding and flexible personality. Empathic teachers may be more likely to help your child in times of difficulty. Many colleges publish course guides containing teacher ratings or make them available in the advising offices for each major to help make these decisions.

Requesting Accommodations

If there are specific ideas that could make the college experience more comfortable or less intimidating for your child, most colleges will gladly make accommodations to assist your child. Examples of accommodations that might be helpful for individuals with ASD include being excused from group projects, receiving preferential seating to suit any auditory or visual sensitivity, and receiving advance notification for changes in schedule. Visual thinkers might ask professors to provide extra visual aids to help them process lectures and course materials. Students with motor coordination difficulties might request extended time on written exams, oral exams, or the option of using a laptop or a tape recorder for note taking. Many colleges offer note-taking services to individuals with cognitive or physical characteristics that make note taking difficult.

Planning a Class Schedule

In planning a schedule, it's always better to start with too few classes than too many. For some students with ASD, the transition to college is so challenging that a full course load would be overwhelming. Starting off slowly and building to a full schedule provides time to adjust to the many changes that college life entails. This will also provide your child with more time to complete work and to devote time to establishing social contacts and planning and engaging in social activities. As you help your child plan a schedule, keep in mind your child's sleeping habits. Try to avoid classes scheduled for an hour of the day when she is typically asleep or groggy. Keep a visual schedule posted in your child's room so she has a handy visual reminder of the times and locations of each class. Unlike high school, during college students are likely to have blocks of free time during the day. For individuals with ASD who thrive on structure and routine, it is important to block these times out on the calendar and specify a designated purpose, such as study time, leisure time, or physical exercise. This added structure and predictability can make college life more comfortable for many people with ASD and can reduce anxiety associated with transitions and changes in schedules.

Monitoring Deadlines

Keep a portable academic calendar with plenty of writing space to mark down homework due dates as well as dates related to registration and class drop deadlines. Encourage your child to check this calendar each morning to have a clear idea of the schedule for the day as well as any upcoming deadlines. Share important deadlines with your child's support people so that they can help him remember. Automated reminders on electronic calendars or mobile devices can also help your child keep track of deadlines and schedules.

Promoting Study Skills

Consistency is crucial to good study habits. Again, planning specific blocks of study time and writing them into a schedule helps students remember to study and gives them a finite goal. These study sessions should be planned for a time of day when your child feels productive and alert. She should find a "study spot" in a library, student center, or computer lab that reliably offers peace and quiet. Students should experiment with different environments to find the type that best suits their own style. For example, some students might feel more comfortable in a dimly lit space with materials scattered around them, while others might prefer a bright, highly organized study spot. Within study sessions, your child might prefer to devote the entire time to one subject or to study several different subjects. If your child prefers the latter approach, it can be helpful to structure her time so that favorite subjects are studied last. This helps motivate your child to persevere through other topics and ensures that more challenging subjects will be addressed while energy is high and attention is most focused. Campus study centers or books on study skills can help out by providing study tips that are applicable to all students, including those with ASD. Most colleges, in their center for students with disabilities, offer some sort of assistance to help students in the domain of organizational skills.

Promoting Social Opportunities

College will provide your adult child with numerous opportunities to further develop his social skills. There are many settings in college where social skills are taught at a more academic level. For example, classes in speech communication and drama emphasize how best to communicate, how to convey emotion, and how to read other people's response to you. Sociology and psychology classes can provide insight into the way others work and the "rules" underlying human behavior. An abundance of special interest groups, ranging from rock group fan clubs to star-gazing societies, provide opportunities for socialization within the comfort of an area of interest. Responding to the increasing presence of students with ASD on college campuses, the administrative offices or student bodies of many colleges are developing ASD friendship or support groups.

Living Arrangements

Some families prefer to have their adult child with ASD continue to live with them. Others, for various reasons, want their adult child to live in the community, in which case several different options are available. Some adults with high-functioning ASD are quite nervous about and uncomfortable with this idea, but many others want this opportunity. Many young adults see it as a way to "normalize" their experience by reaching the same milestone as their siblings and peers. A wealth of practical matters, such as housework, household maintenance, cooking, shopping, transportation, and bill paying, can make independent living difficult for individuals with ASD, however. Your adult child's ability to accomplish these kinds of tasks *on her own, with minimal supervision,* needs to be considered when selecting the most appropriate living situation. If you're concerned about your child's ability to live independently, start at a more supported level; preparing your child for increased independence can make the transition less overwhelming. Remember, too, that none of these decisions is permanent.

Most outside-the-family-home living arrangements are accessed through state agencies (with the exception of the first one we discuss below, independent living). The first step in finding these living arrangements is determining your child's eligibility for these state services. The name of the agency that provides residential services differs from state to state, but it is usually the same agency that provides respite, vocational-rehabilitation, and other services to people with disabilities. They often have names like the "Division of Developmental Disabilities" or the "Department of Developmental Services." Many states now have specific divisions focused on provision of services for individuals with ASD. The doctor who diagnosed your child, your state autism society, or even a local pediatrician or psychologist may be helpful in determining the correct contact. This agency should have a designated webpage linked from your state government website. When you and your child begin the evaluation process that determines eligibility for services, be sure to emphasize the limitations your child has in accomplishing activities of daily life *independently*. Sometimes people with ASD are denied state-funded disability services because their level of handicap is perceived as minimal compared to those with severe ASD or mental retardation. But if you stress that your child cannot do necessary activities like feeding himself (since this requires shopping, money handling, and other skills he may not have) or engage in daily hygiene unless someone assists him, he will be more likely to be eligible for the residential assistance options we describe below.

Independent Living

Independent living refers to your adult child living on her own without professional or significant family support. Independent living might, however, include a roommate who could be a source of support. For adults with ASD who are living independently, support people are especially crucial. Your child should have "go-to" people who live nearby and can be contacted for various kinds of support. People with ASD who are able to live independently may still need professional help in areas that involve crucial decision making, such as selecting homeowner's or renter's insurance or life insurance, or in financial matters. Based on her firsthand experience living as an adult with ASD, Liane Willey suggests some organizational strategies to help people with ASD who are living independently. She also recommends that a support person help your adult child get these strategies up and running.

• Sort mail into color-coded bins according to type, such as magazines, bills, correspondence, and so on. Set a specific time on a certain day of the week to go through the bills bin and pay those that are due. This kind of structure and routine helps to ensure that bills will not be overlooked and deadlines will not be missed. You can work with your child to set up electronic auto-pay arrangement for bills so that it is not necessary to take action each month. Although this reduces independence, you could also pay his bills yourself by accessing his electronic accounts.

• Maintain color-coded paper or computer files for documenting and storing information involving credit cards, automobile maintenance and insurance, checkbooks, family wills and related legal documents, financial records, home or life insurance, household appliance instructions and warranty information, and health records. Software programs, such as Evernote, enable a person to simply photograph important documents (for example, with a mobile phone camera) to have the text recognized and placed in an easily searchable database. Such programs use ease of search to reduce the need for consistent organization, which may be beneficial to individuals who struggle with executive function.

• Use an electronic calendar to record all household responsibilities or related appointments on a weekly or monthly schedule. By using Internet "cloud" support, this information can then be present and modifiable on the devices of multiple people, such as both you and your child. It may also be helpful to print monthly or weekly calendars and put them in a prominent place around your house. Although a portable calendar is convenient because it can travel with your child, it may lack the visual salience of a large calendar and is unlikely to be useful unless your child regularly accesses it.

• For important one-time reminders, stick adhesive-backed notes on the bathroom mirror so they will be impossible to miss during the course of the day or when getting ready in the morning. Again, alarms on mobile devices can be used as reminders.

• Location-based reminders on mobile devices can also be helpful. For example, your child might set her phone to remind her to take her laptop case when she leaves the house in the morning.

Tools for Growing Independence

- "Go-to" people in different settings: school, work, sports, clubs, social arenas.
- Disclosure cards or a rehearsed script.
- Explicit rules for romantic and sexual behavior.
- Visual calendars and automated or location-based reminders on mobile devices.
- Exploration of autism, self-identity, and self-acceptance through books, support groups, and online communities.
- Medication or cognitive-behavioral therapy for mood and anxiety problems.
- Educational accommodations in college.
- Organization systems for paperwork or use of database software that can scan images and recognize text.
- Online grocery ordering and delivery services.
- Individualized transition plan to college or workplace.
- Online job procurement and employment opportunities.
- Job coaches.
- Residential living options through state agencies that determine eligibility.

For many people with ASD, overwhelming sensory stimulation and crowds of people can make shopping extremely difficult. Thanks to catalogs and web shopping, your child may not have to leave home to obtain many items, including groceries. When your child does have to run errands or go shopping, ask a support person to go along. Or an adult child who finds certain errands less intimidating or enjoyable can offer to do those for a support person in exchange for the support person's taking over more challenging tasks for the person with ASD.

Supervised Group Living

Another residential option that provides more support than independent living is supervised group living. One type of supervised group living is a group home, which is a residential facility for several individuals with disabilities. Group homes are usually houses in residential neighborhoods staffed by trained professionals who assist residents in areas like personal care, cooking, and housekeeping. Since group homes may serve individuals with various disabilities, it may be advantageous to seek one that specializes in ASD.

A second type of supervised group living is a supervised apartment. In a supervised apartment, an individual lives with fewer people, and professionals visit only a couple of times per week. This arrangement affords the residents more independence and greater responsibility and is therefore often an excellent means of preparation for independent living.

Skill Development Homes

In skill development homes residents live with a family in their dwelling and the family receives funding from the agency responsible for the individual's care. In this arrangement, the family members have been trained to work with people with ASD and can be expected to provide assistance and instruction in self-care skills and housekeeping.

Employment

Finding appropriate employment is crucial in many straightforward practical ways, but it is also an important means of boosting a person's self-esteem and providing social opportunities. You will want to begin planning for your child's eventual employment well before your child will actually approach the job market, probably as he enters adolescence. This provides time to prepare your child for the challenges of the workplace and to help him develop requisite marketable skills. For many individuals with ASD, preparation for employment will be a part of the Individualized Transition Plan described above.

Employment Options

There are several different types of employment settings, discussed here in descending order of amount of independence and self-sufficiency required.

Competitive Employment

Competitive employment refers to the typical type of job that most people apply and compete for. Such jobs do not usually offer support for your adult child as part of the work environment, so they represent the most independent option of those we've listed. Some people with ASD succeed in competitive employment, especially when they opt for jobs that play to their strengths (see below) or minimize the amount of interpersonal contact required. Also within the domain of competitive employment is self-employment, or running your own business. Although this can mean increased organizational demands, it also allows your adult child to make the rules and set things up to suit his or her own preferences or needs. It can also offer an opportunity to tailor employment to the person's own interests. Some people with ASD have chosen the option of running a business over the Internet since it may reduce direct interpersonal contact and social demands. One young man we know ran a website that brokered the sale of used books.

Supported Employment

"Supported employment" refers to a system of supports that allow individuals with disabilities to obtain paid employment in the community. Supported employment includes individual placement, clustered or enclave models, mobile crews, and the entrepreneurial model. "Individual placement" refers to a model in which a specific job is developed for a specific person by a job coach. This professional also works with the individual on the job to help her develop the necessary skills to do the job well. The "cluster," or "enclave placement," model is similar, but the job coach works with a group of people at the employment site. Mobile crews also consist of a small group of individuals and one job coach, but they work at different job sites and for different employers (for example, cleaning homes or offices in the community). In the entrepreneurial model, a small business is developed to employ persons with disabilities. At Division TEACCH, the center for individuals with ASD in North Carolina (described in Chapter 4), they have developed several businesses that are staffed by people with ASD, including one that makes the materials needed for a test kit used by professionals to measure symptoms of ASD.

Secure Employment

"Secure employment" refers to a facility-based employment placement in which an individual is guaranteed a job, usually doing basic tasks in a structured setting. In a secure employment setting, individuals also receive work skills and behavior training to prepare them for more independent and competitive work environments.

Sheltered Workshops

Like secure employment, sheltered workshops are employment services associated with training agencies that employ many individuals with disabilities. However, placement in a sheltered workshop setting may not provide sufficient training for individuals to progress toward more independent employment settings. For this reason, secure employment settings are generally preferable to sheltered workshops.

Choosing a Job

An appropriate job should capitalize on the strengths of your son or daughter in terms of both preferences and natural abilities. We have discussed the passion and conviction with which many people with ASD pursue their interests and the knowledge that they can accumulate about their preferred subject matter. Applying this enthusiasm and ability in the workplace is an ideal means of helping people with ASD to succeed in employment. For example, a person who is fascinated by bus routes and schedules would be a natural candidate for a job with a transportation department. As we described in Chapter 5, a person interested in history might enjoy working in an archives department. Of course, there is more to successful employment than simply being interested in the job responsibilities. However, a passion for the subject matter addressed in the job can provide excellent motivation for confronting the challenges it presents.

Consider jobs that involve a high level of routine and order. "Rule-governed" people may be more likely to succeed in jobs that have clearly defined rules, procedures, or routines, such as in a payroll office, a library, or a business that performs data entry. Jobs that require less direct interaction with others or that can be done through telecommuting or consist of primarily computer-oriented responsibilities may be appropriate for individuals who feel uncomfortable in interpersonal interactions.

Rupert, an adult with high-functioning ASD, worked in a small office building and delivered the mail to the individuals who worked there. He liked routine and was aware that he was able to perform better and more comfortably when things were as he expected them to be. With his supervisor, he set up a daily schedule and mail route. Sticking to this schedule and having an available "consultant" should things change helped Rupert to succeed in the workplace.

Look for job opportunities that capitalize on your child's strong visualization or memory skills. A great example of tailoring a job to a strength in visual thinking is Temple Grandin's remarkable ability to use her visual mind to construct and test cow-handling facilities. Employment opportunities that feature tangible tasks, such as cooking, organizing, or computer programming, seem naturally suited to people who tend to think in visual terms. Jobs that require knowledge of lots of specific details or facts, such as working with inventory or in a library, can be a good match for adults with ASD who have a strong rote memory.

A useful place to begin is to compose a list of your child's likes and preferences. Think creatively. For example, an interest in crafts might be turned into a website where decorative items are sold. An interest in baseball could translate into trading and selling baseball memorabilia. It is important to consider such things as level of interpersonal contact, physical requirements, sensory stimulation and level of activity in the workplace, and the flexibility of the work schedule. Think about whether your child would enjoy or be able to tolerate these aspects of the work setting. Appropriate jobs might include engineer, computer programmer, florist, medical transcriber, artist/craftsman, musician, factory worker, architect, electronic repairperson, librarian, antiques/collectibles trader, and archivist. This is not by any means an exhaustive list. It is intended to provide a range of options, from those requiring advanced degrees to those that can be obtained fresh from high school, that all require good visual skills, involve high degrees of routine and order, and are more hands-on than abstract in nature.

There are also computerized resources to assist with job procurement. The Attainment Company (*www.attainmentcompany.com*) markets software for this purpose. At their website, you can peruse software that is designed to help you work through your child's characteristics and how they match up with job requirements and social skills associated with employment. Many advocacy groups, such as Autism Speaks, offer webpages with specific information on employment and transition strategies as well as actual supported job opportunities.

Especially for a first job, it is essential to pick one with a high probability of success. This will help your adult child adapt to the experience of working while reducing his worry about failure. It will also give your child a chance to experience firsthand the reinforcing properties of succeeding in the workplace and earning a salary.

Interviewing

Interviewing is a crucial skill for all job applicants, so it's important to work specifically on this skill with your adult child. Make a specific and concrete list of inappropriate and appropriate behaviors. If you know of any inappropriate habits your child has, such as clearing her throat loudly or picking at scabs, include them on the list. Write out a script that includes likely questions that the interviewer will ask and appropriate responses. Practice this script with your child using role playing to help your child memorize answers and to increase his or her comfort in this type of situation. Be sure to pay attention to aspects of nonverbal communication in both the interviewer and your child. Important aspects of nonverbal behavior to include are greetings and good-byes, eye contact, voice volume and pace, display of emotion or anxiety, dressing appropriately, appearing well groomed, and proper posture. Emphasize to your child how important it will be to attend to everything the interviewer says during the interview. For more information about the types of behaviors that are helpful during interviews, consult a book addressing work application and interviewing particulars.

Once your child has practiced these skills and feels comfortable role-playing them with a support person, it can be helpful to do a "throw-away" interview. Apply for a job that will involve interviewing but is undesirable or in a less preferred field. Scheduling an interview with less riding on the line will give your child the opportunity to practice interviewing skills in a real setting. Doing so can reduce her anxiety and the feeling of total unfamiliarity when your child later interviews for a job she genuinely desires.

Workplace Accommodations

Before you can ask for accommodations in the workplace, your child must decide whether to disclose information about his diagnosis. Accommodations can be made in a number of areas. Adjustments in workspace may help with sensory or motor characteristics. Use visual approaches to teach job skills. Creating visual "supports" for the workplace, such as a written set of instructions or picture diagrams of the finished product, can be beneficial to visual thinkers. It may also be important to ask for special considerations if work requirements entail cooperating in groups. Scheduling accommodations could help increase routine or decrease unpredictability in work demands. Finally, it may be important to work out a plan with an employer for management and resolution of any crises that may develop on the job.

A Final Word

Our goal in this book has been to help you give your child the best chance possible for a full and happy life. As your understanding of the strengths associated with ASD grows, so will your ability to conquer its challenges. And as you overcome the difficulties that your child's disorder presents, you will be more able to celebrate the gifts and joys that your unique son or daughter brings to your life. The challenges may never entirely go away, but with your understanding and proper treatment as early as possible, your child and family can expect lots of improvement over the years. The more we learn about high-functioning ASD, the more likely it is that your child will, in fact, lead a full and happy life.

Resources

Books on ASD

General Information on Autism Spectrum Disorder

Attwood, Tony. (2007). *The complete guide to Asperger's syndrome*. London: Kingsley.

Baron-Cohen, Simon. (2008). *Autism and Asperger syndrome: The facts*. Oxford, UK: Oxford University Press.

Romanowski Bashe, Patricia & Kirby, Barbara. (2010). *The OASIS guide to Asperger syndrome: Completely revised and updated: Advice, support, insight, and inspiration*. New York: Random House.

Bernier, Raphael, & Gerdts, Jennifer. (2010). *Autism spectrum disorders: A reference handbook*. Santa Barbara, CA: ABC-CLIO.

Chawarska, Katarzyna, Klin, Ami, & Volkmar, Fred R. (Eds.). (2010). *Autism spectrum disorders in infants and toddlers*. New York: Guilford Press.

McPartland, James C., Klin, Ami, & Volkmar, Fred R. (Eds.). (2014). *Asperger syndrome: Assessing and treating high-functioning autism spectrum disorders* (2nd ed.). New York: Guilford Press.

Mesibov, Gary B., Shea, Victoria, & Schopler, Eric. (2004). *The TEACCH approach to autism spectrum disorders*. New York: Springer.

Sicile-Kira, Chantal. (2014). *Autism spectrum disorders: The complete guide to understanding autism* (rev. ed.). New York: Penguin.

Siegel, Bryna. (2007). *Helping children with autism learn: Treatment approaches for parents and professionals.* Oxford, UK: Oxford University Press.

Parenting, Family Issues, and Parents' Perspectives

Brooks, Robert, & Goldstein, Sam. (2012). *Raising resilient children with autism spectrum disorders: Strategies for helping them maximize their strengths, cope with adversity, and develop a social mindset.* New York: McGraw-Hill.

Cook O'Toole, Jennifer. (2013). *Asperkids: An insider's guide to loving, understanding, and teaching children with Asperger's syndrome.* London: Kingsley.

Doyle, Barbara T., & Iland, Emily Doyle. (2004). *Autism spectrum disorders from A to Z.* Arlington, TX: Future Horizons.

Fling, Echo. (2000). *Eating an artichoke: A mother's perspective on Asperger syndrome.* London: Kingsley.

Harris, Sandra L., & Glasberg, Beth A. (2012). *Siblings of children with autism: A guide for families.* Bethesda, MD: Woodbine House.

Hughes-Lynch, Claire. (2010). *Children with high-functioning autism: A parent's guide.* Austin, TX: Prufrock Press.

LeComer, Laurie F. (2006). *A parent's guide to developmental delays: Recognizing and coping with missed milestones in speech, movement, learning and other areas.* Bellevue, WA: Perigee.

Naseef, Robert A. (2013). *Autism in the family: Caring and coping together.* Baltimore: Brookes.

Park, Clara. (2002). *Exiting nirvana: A daughter's life with autism.* Boston: Back Bay Books.

Rapee, Ronald M., Wignall, Ann, Spence, Susan H., Cobham, Vanessa, & Lyneham, Heidi. (2010). *Helping your anxious child: A step-by-step guide for parents.* Oakland, CA: New Harbinger.

Rosenblatt, Alan, & Carbone, Paul S. (Eds.). (2012). *Autism spectrum disorders: What every parent needs to know.* Washington, DC: American Academy of Pediatrics.

Schilling, Shonda. (2010). *The best kind of different: Our family's journey with Asperger's syndrome.* New York: HarperCollins.

Volkmar, Fred R., & Wiesner, Lisa A. (2009). *A practical guide to autism:*

What every parent, family member, and teacher needs to know. New York: Wiley.

Willey, Liane. (2001). *Asperger syndrome in the family: Redefining normal.* London: Kingsley.

Education and Related Issues

Chalfant, Anne M. (2011). *Managing anxiety in people with autism: A treatment guide for parents, teachers, and mental health professionals.* Bethesda, MD: Woodbine House.

Cumine, Val, Dunlop, Julia, & Stevenson, Gill. (2009). *Asperger syndrome: A practical guide for teachers.* London: Fulton.

Eason, Anne I., & Whitebread, Kathleen. (2006). *IEP and inclusion tips for parents and teachers (handout version).* Verona, WI: Attainment Company.

Freedman, Sarita. (2010). *Developing college skills in students with autism and Asperger's syndrome.* London: Kingsley.

Gibb, Gordon, & Dyches, Tina Taylor. (2007). *Guide to writing quality individualized education programs (IEPs): What's best for students?* Boston: Allyn & Bacon.

Hodgdon, Linda A. (2011). *Visual strategies for improving communication: Practical supports for school and home.* Troy, MI: QuickRoberts.

Lentz, Kirby. (2005). *Hopes and dreams: An IEP guide for parents of children with autism spectrum disorders.* Lenexa, KS: Autism Asperger Publishing Company.

Moyes, Rebecca, & Moreno, Susan. (2001). *Incorporating social goals in the classroom: A guide for teachers and parents of children with high-functioning autism and Asperger syndrome.* London: Kingsley.

Myles, Brenda Smith, Adreon, Diane, & Gitlitz, Dena. (2006). *Simple strategies that work: Helpful hints for all educators of students with Asperger syndrome, high-functioning autism, and related disabilities.* Lenexa, KS: Autism Asperger Publishing Company.

Reaven, Judy, Blakely-Smith, Audrey, & Nichols, Shana. (2011). *Facing your fears.* Baltimore: Brookes.

Siegel, Lawrence. (2011). *The complete IEP guide: How to advocate for your special ed child* (7th ed.). Berkeley, CA: Nolo Press.

Silverman, Stephan M., & Weinfeld, Rich. (2007). *School success for kids with Asperger's syndrome: A practical guide for parents and teachers.* Austin, TX: Prufrock Press.

Tanguay, Pamela, & Rourke, Byron. (2001). *Nonverbal learning disabilities at home: A parent's guide.* London: Kingsley.

Wright, Peter W. D., & Darr Wright, Pamela. (2007). *Wrightslaw: Special education law* (2nd ed.). Hartfield, VA: Harbor House Law Press.

Wright, Peter W. D., Darr Wright, Pamela, & Webb O'Connor, Sandra. (2010). *Wrightslaw: All about IEPs.* Hartfield, VA: Harbor House Law Press.

Social Skills Training and Other Social Interventions

Bellini, Scott. (2006). *Building social relationships: A systematic approach to teaching social interaction skills to children and adolescents with autism spectrum disorders and other social difficulties.* Lenexa, KS: Autism Asperger Publishing Company.

Bondy, Andy, & Weiss, Mary Jane. (2013). *Teaching social skills to people with autism: Best practices in individualizing interventions.* Bethesda, MD: Woodbine House.

Elman, Natalie Madorsky, & Kennedy-Moore, Eileen. (2003). *The unwritten rules of friendship: Simple strategies to help your child make friends.* New York: Little, Brown and Company.

Garcia-Winner, Michelle. (2002). *Inside out: What makes a person with social cognitive deficits tick?* San Jose, CA: Winner Publications (*www.socialthinking.com*).

Gray, Carol. (2010). *The new social story book, revised and expanded 10th anniversary edition.* Arlington, TX: Future Horizons.

Ingersoll, Brooke, & Dvortcsak, Anna. (2010). *Teaching social communication to children with autism: A manual for parents.* New York: Guilford Press.

Koenig, Kathleen. (2012). *Practical social skills for autism spectrum disorders: Designing child-specific interventions.* New York: Norton.

Laugeson, Elizabeth A., & Frankel, Fred. (2010). *Social skills for teenagers with developmental and autism spectrum disorders: The PEERS treatment manual.* New York: Routledge.

McClannahan, Lynn E., & Krantz, Patricia. (2010). *Activity schedules for children with autism: Teaching independent behavior.* Bethesda, MD: Woodbine House.

Tubbs, Janet. (2007). *Creative therapy for children with autism, ADD, and Asperger's: Using artistic creativity to reach, teach, and touch our children.* Garden City Park, NY: Square One Publishers.

Teasing and Bullying

Dubin, Nick. (2007). *Asperger Syndrome and bullying: Strategies and solutions.* London: Kingsley.

Garrity, Carla, Baris, Mitchell, & Porter, William. (2000). *Bully-proofing your child: A parent's guide.* Longmont, CO: Sopris West.

Garrity, Carla, Jens, Kathryn, Porter, William, Sager, Nancy, & Short-Camilli, Cam. (2000). *Bully-proofing your school: A comprehensive approach for elementary schools.* Longmont, CO: Sopris West.

Garrity, Carla, Porter, William, & Baris, Mitchell. (2000). *Bully-proofing your child: First aid for hurt feelings.* Longmont, CO: Sopris West.

Heinrichs, Rebekah. (2003). *Perfect targets: Asperger syndrome and bullying—Practical solutions for surviving the social world.* Lenexa, KS: Autism Asperger Publishing Company.

Developing Self-Identity

Faherty, Catherine. (2000). *Asperger's . . . What does it mean to me?: A workbook explaining self-awareness and life lessons to the child or youth with high-functioning autism or Asperger's.* Arlington, TX: Future Horizons.

Shore, Stephen M. (2004). *Ask and tell: Self-advocacy and disclosure for people on the autism spectrum.* Lenexa, KS: Autism Asperger Publishing Company.

Vermeulen, Peter. (2008). *I am special: Introducing children and young people to their autism spectrum disorder.* London: Kingsley.

Behavioral and Sensory Issues

Baker, Bruce L., & Brightman, Alan J. (2003). *Steps to independence: A skills training guide for parents and teachers of children with special needs.* Baltimore: Brookes.

Biel, Lindsey, & Peake, Nancy. (2009). *Raising a sensory smart child: The definitive handbook for helping your child with sensory processing issues.* New York: Penguin.

Durand, V. Mark. (2013). *Sleep better!: A guide to improving sleep for children with special needs.* Baltimore: Brookes.

Kranowitz, Carol Stock. (2006). *The out of sync child: Recognizing and coping with sensory integration dysfunction.* Bellevue, WA: Perigee.

Myles, Brenda Smith, Cook, Katherine, & Miller, Louann. (2002). *Asperger syndrome and sensory issues: Practical solutions for making sense of the world.* Lenexa, KS: Autism Asperger Publishing Company.

Myles, Brenda Smith, & Southwick, Jack. (2005). *Asperger syndrome and difficult moments: Practical solutions for tantrums, rage, and meltdowns.* Lenexa, KS: Autism Asperger Publishing Company.

O'Neill, Robert, Albin, Richard, Storey, Keith, Horner, Robert, & Sprague, Jeffrey. (2014). *Functional assessment and program development for problem behavior: A practical handbook.* Pacific Grove, CA: Brookes/Cole.

Preschool Treatment Models

Ball, James. (2008). *Early intervention and autism: Real-life questions, real-life answers.* Arlington, TX: Future Horizons.

Bricker, Diane. (2004). *An activity-based approach to early intervention.* Baltimore: Brookes.

Greenspan, Stanley, & Wieder, Serena. (2009). *Engaging autism: Using the Floortime approach to help children relate, communicate, and think.* Cambridge, MA: Perseus Press.

Harris, Sandra L., & Weiss, Mary Jane. (2007). *Right from the start: Behavioral intervention for young children with autism: A guide for parents and professionals.* Bethesda, MD: Woodbine House.

Rogers, Sally J., Dawson, Geraldine, & Vismara, Laurie A. (2012). *An early start for your child with autism: Using everyday activities to help kids connect, communicate, and learn.* New York: Guilford Press.

Rogers, Sally J., & Dawson, Geraldine. (2009). *Early Start Denver Model for young children with autism: Promoting language, learning, and engagement.* New York: Guilford Press.

Sher, Barbara. (2009). *Early intervention games: Fun, joyful ways to develop social and motor skills in children with autism spectrum or sensory processing disorders.* New York: Wiley.

Adulthood and Employment

Bissonnette, Barbara. (2013). *The complete guide to getting a job for people with Asperger's syndrome: Find the right career and get hired.* London: Kingsley.

Endow, Judy, & Myles, Brenda Smith. (2013). *The hidden curriculum of getting and keeping a job: Navigating the social landscape of employment: A guide for individuals with autism spectrum and other social-cognitive challenges.* Lenexa, KS: Autism Asperger Publishing Company.

Howlin, Patricia. (2004). *Autism and Asperger syndrome: Preparing for adulthood.* London: Routledge.

Krouk-Gordon, Dafna, & Jackins, Barbara D. (2013). *Moving out: A family guide to residential planning for adults with disabilities.* Bethesda, MD: Woodbine House.

Meyer, Roger N., & Attwood, Tony. (2001). *Asperger syndrome employment workbook: An employment workbook for adults with Asperger syndrome.* London: Kingsley.

Sicile-Kira, Chantal, & Sicile-Kira, Jeremy. (2012). *A full life with autism: From learning to forming relationships to achieving independence.* New York: Palgrave Macmillan.

Volkmar, Fred, Reichow, Brian, & McPartland, James C. (2014). *Adolescents and adults with autism spectrum disorder.* New York: Springer.

Wehman, Paul, Smith, Marcia, & Schall, Carol. (2008). *Autism and the transition to adulthood: Success beyond the classroom.* Baltimore, MD: Brookes.

Personal Accounts

Cook O'Toole, Jennifer. (2012). *Asperkids secret book of social rules: The handbook of not-so-obvious social guidelines for tweens and teens with Asperger syndrome.* London: Kingsley.

Grandin, Temple. (2006). *Thinking in pictures, expanded edition: My life with autism.* New York: Vintage Books.

Grandin, Temple, & Panek, Richard. (2013). *The autistic brain: Thinking across the spectrum.* Boston: Houghton Mifflin Harcourt.

Jackson, Luke. (2002). *Freaks, geeks, and Asperger syndrome: A user guide to adolescence.* London: Kingsley.

Olinkiewicz, Alex, & O'Connell, Richard. (2012). *In my mind: A journey through my life with Asperger's/autism.* Charleston, SC: CreateSpace Independent Publishing Platform.

O'Neal, Jaylon V. (2013). *Autism: In my own words.* Bloomington, IN: AuthorHouse.

Pulver, Marc William. (2012). *Living life with autism: The world through my eyes.* Indianapolis, IN: Dog Ear.

Robison, John Elder. (2008). *Look me in the eye: My life with Asperger's.* New York: Three Rivers Press.

Software and Applications

AppyMall: Apps for kids
www.appymall.com

Attainment Company
www.attainmentcompany.com

AutisMate
http://autismate.com/AutisMate-Comprehensive-App-For-Autism-With-Visual-Supports/

Autism Speaks App Resource List
www.autismspeaks.org/autism-apps

Choiceworks
www.beevisual.com

Do2Learn
www.do2learn.com

Emotion and Feelings—Autism
https://play.google.com/store/apps/details?id=com.TouchAutism.
EmotionsFeelings&hl=en

HandHold Adaptive (iPrompts, StoryMaker, SpeechPrompts)
www.handholdadaptive.com

I Get It!: Educational Applications for iPhone, iPad, and iPodTouch
http://igetitapps.com

The iMums: Reviews of Apps for Children
www.theimum.com

iTubeList
www.itubelist.net

Kid in Story
http://locomotivelabs.com

Laureate Learning Systems
www.laureatelearning.com

LocuTour Multimedia
www.learningfundamentals.com

Mayer-Johnson
www.mayer-johnson.com

My PlayHome
www.myplayhomeapp.com

Pictello
www.assistiveware.com/product/pictello

The Planner Guide
www.autismspeaks.org/autism-apps/planner-guide

Scientific Learning
www.scilearn.com

Smart Apps for Special Needs
www.smartappsforspecialneeds.com

Special Education Apps
www.a4cwsn.com

Special Needs Apps
www.friendshipcircle.org/apps

Technology in (SPL) Education
www.techinspecialed.com

Touch Autism
http://touchautism.com/app/autism-apps

Websites for ASD Resources

Asperger Autism Spectrum Education Network (ASPEN)
www.aspennj.org

Association for Science in Autism Treatment
www.asatonline.org

Autism Consortium
www.autismconsortium.org

Autism Link
www.autismlink.com

Autism Research Institute
www.autism.com

Autism-Resources
www.autism-resources.com

Autism Science Foundation
www.autismsciencefoundation.org

Autism Shop: Products for Children and Adults with Autism
www.autismshop.com

Autism Society of America
www.autism-society.org

Autism Speaks
www.autismspeaks.org

Autism Spectrum Resource Center
www.autismconnecticut.org

Autism Today
www.autismtoday.com

Children's Friendship Training
www.semel.ucla.edu/socialskills

Families for Early Autism Treatment
www.feat.org

First Signs
www.firstsigns.org

Future Horizons
www.fhautism.com

Generation Rescue
www.generationrescue.org

Global and Regional Asperger Syndrome Partnership
www.grasp.org/main

Global Autism Collaboration
www.globalautismcollaboration.com

The Help Group
www.thehelpgroup.org/autism-spectrum-disorders-schools-programs

Interactive Autism Network
www.iancommunity.org

MIND Institute
www.ucdmc.ucdavis.edu/mindinstitute

National Autistic Society
www.nas.org.uk

Online Asperger Syndrome Information & Support Services for Autism & Asperger Syndrome (OASIS)
www.aspergersyndrome.org

Oops . . . Wrong Planet Syndrome
www.wrongplanet.net

Sibling Support
www.siblingsupport.org/sibshops

Simons Foundation Autism Research Initiative
https://sfari.org

Special Needs.com
www.SpecialNeeds.com

Websites for Adults with ASD

Asperger Adults
www.aspergeradults.ca

Autism Journals: Asperger's Pride Websites
www.rdos.net/eng

Autism Network International
autreat.com

The Global and Regional Asperger Syndrome Partnership
http://grasp.org

Websites for Families and Friends

Camphill Communities
www.camphill.org

Families of Adults Affected by Asperger's Syndrome (FAAAS)
www.faaas.org

Family Support
www.patientcenters.com/autism/news/stress_family.html

Planned Lifetime Advocacy Network
www.plan.ca

Sibling Support Project
www.siblingsupport.org

Unlocking Autism Parent 2 Parent Network
www.unlockingautism.org

Websites for Associated Learning Disabilities

The ARC
www.thearc.org

Children and Adults with Attention-Deficit/Hyperactivity Disorder
www.chadd.org

Learning Disabilities Association of America
www.ldanatl.org

Learning Disabilities Online
www.ldonline.org

Nonverbal Learning Disability Line
www.nldline.com

Our-Kids: Devoted to Raising Special Kids with Special Needs
www.our-kids.org

Academic Medical Centers and Clinics

Boston University Autism Center
www.bu.edu/autism/current-research/autism-center-of-excellence

Carolina Institute for Developmental Disabilities
www.cidd.unc.edu

Center for Children with Special Needs
www.autismct.com

Center for Excellence in Autism Research at the University of
Pittsburgh
www.wpic.pitt.edu/research/cefar

Children's Evaluation and Rehabilitation Center at the Albert Einstein
College of Medicine
www.einstein.yu.edu/centers/childrens-evaluation-rehabilitation

Children's Hospital of Philadelphia Center for Autism Research
www.research.chop.edu/programs/car

Cody Center for Autism and Developmental Disabilities
www.stonybrookmedicalcenter.org/codycenter

Douglass Developmental Disabilities Center at Rutgers
http://dddc.rutgers.edu

A. J. Drexel Autism Institute
www.drexel.edu/autisminstitute

Duke Center for Autism and Brain Development
Duke University School of Medicine
2608 Erwin Road, Suite 300
Durham, NC 27705
919-687-4686, Ext. 240

Indiana Resource Center for Autism
www.iidc.indiana.edu/index.php?pageId=32

Kennedy Krieger Institute
www.autism.kennedykrieger.org/?gclid=CL7Prdq7q70CFQ2hOgodoiwAJw

Lurie Center for Autism at MassGeneral Hospital for Children
www.massgeneral.org/children/services/treatmentprograms.aspx?id=1614

Marcus Autism Center
www.marcus.org

New York-Presbyterian Center for Autism and the Developing Brain
http://nyp.org/autism

Rush University Medical Center Autism Resource Center
www.rush.edu/rumc/page-1213718660256.html

Seattle Children's Autism Center
www.seattlechildrens.org/clinics-programs/autism-center

Seaver Autism Center at Mount Sinai
http://icahn.mssm.edu/research/centers/seaver-autism-center

Southwest Autism Research and Resource Center
www.autismcenter.org

UC Davis MIND Institute
www.ucdmc.ucdavis.edu/mindinstitute

UCLA Center for Autism Research and Treatment (CART)
www.semel.ucla.edu/autism

UCLA Peers Clinic
www.semel.ucla.edu/peers

UCSB Koegel Autism Center
http://education.ucsb.edu/autism

UCSF Autism and Neurodevelopment Program
https://psych.ucsf.edu/autism

University of Cambridge Autism Research Center
www.autismresearchcentre.com

University of Louisville Autism Center
https://louisville.edu/autism

University of Miami Center for Autism and Related Disabilities
www.umcard.org

University of Michigan Autism and Communication Disorders Center
http://webservices.itcs.umich.edu/drupal/chgddev/umacc

University of North Carolina at Chapel Hill Division TEACCH
http://teacch.com

University of North Dakota Global Rural Autism Asperger Information Network (GRAAIN)
www.und.nodak.edu/org/graain

UT Southwestern Autism Center
www.utsouthwestern.edu/education/medicschool/departments/psychiatry/autism/index.html

University of Washington Autism Center
http://depts.washington.edu/uwautism/index.php

Vanderbilt Treatment and Research Institute for Autism Spectrum Disorders
http://kc.vanderbilt.edu/triad

Virginia Tech Center for Autism Research
www.vtcar.science.vt.edu

Waisman Center at the University of Wisconsin–Madison
www.waisman.wisc.edu/clinics-asd-dd.htm

Yale Child Study Center Autism Program
www.autism.fm

References

American Psychiatric Association. (1994). *Diagnostic and statistical manual of mental disorders* (4th ed.). Washington, DC: Author.

American Psychiatric Association. (2013). *Diagnostic and statistical manual of mental disorders* (5th ed.). Arlington, VA: Author.

Anagnostou, E., & Taylor, M. J. (2011). Review of neuroimaging in autism spectrum disorders: What we have learned and where we go from here. *Molecular Autism, 2*(1), 4.

Asperger, H. (1944/1991). "Autistic psychopathy" in childhood. In U. Frith (Ed.), *Autism and Asperger syndrome* (pp. 37–92). New York: Cambridge University Press.

Bailey, A., Palferman, S., Heavey, L., & LeCouteur, A. (1998). Autism: The phenotype in relatives. *Journal of Autism and Developmental Disorders, 28,* 369–392.

Ballan, M. S. (2012). Parental perspectives of communication about sexuality in families of children with autism spectrum disorders. *Journal of Autism and Developmental Disorders, 42,* 676–684.

Baribeau, D. A., & Anagnostou, E. (2014). An update on medication management of behavioral disorders in autism. *Current Psychiatry Reports, 16*(3), 437.

Baron-Cohen, S. (2000). Is Asperger syndrome/high-functioning autism necessarily a disability? *Development and Psychopathology, 12,* 489–500.

Baron-Cohen, S., Bolton, P., Wheelwright, S., Short, L., Mead, G., Smith, A., et al. (1998). Autism occurs more often in families of physicists, engineers, and mathematicians. *Autism: The International Journal of Research and Practice, 2,* 296–301.

Baron-Cohen, S., Ring, H. A., Wheelwright, S., Bullmore, E., Brammer, M., Simmons, A., et al. (1999). Social intelligence in the normal and autistic brain: An fMRI study. *European Journal of Neuroscience, 11,* 1891–1898.

Bryan, L. C., & Gast, D. L. (2000). Teaching on-task and on-schedule behaviors to high-functioning children with autism via picture activity schedules. *Journal of Autism and Developmental Disorders, 30,* 553–567.

Case-Smith, J., Weaver, L. L., & Fristad, M. A. (2014, January 29). A systematic review of sensory processing interventions for children with autism spectrum disorders. *Autism.* Published online before print: *http://aut.sagepub.com/content/early/2014/01/29/136236131351 7762.full*

Centers for Disease Control and Prevention. (2014). Prevalence of autism spectrum disorders. *MMWR Surveillance Summaries, 63,* 1–24.

Chaste, P., & Leboyer, M. (2012). Autism risk factors: Genes, environment, and gene–environment interactions. *Dialogues in Clinical Neuroscience, 14*(3), 281–292.

Courchesne, E., Pierce, K., Schumann, C. M., Redcay, E., Buckwalter, M. A., Kennedy, D. P., et al. (2007). Mapping early brain development in autism. *Neuron, 56*(2), 399–413.

Courchesne, E., Redcay, E., & Kennedy, D. P. (2004). The autistic brain: Birth through adulthood. *Current Opinions in Neuroscience, 17*(4), 489–496.

Crosland, K., & Dunlap, G. (2012). Effective strategies for the inclusion of children with autism in general education classrooms. *Behavior Modification, 36,* 251–269.

Damasio, A. R., & Maurer, R. G. (1978). A neurological model for childhood autism. *Archives of Neurology, 35,* 777–786.

Dawson, G., & Bernier, R. (2013). A quarter century of progress on the early detection and treatment of autism spectrum disorder. *Developmental Psychopathology, 25,* 1455–1472.

Dawson, G., Carver, L., Meltzoff, A. N., Panagiotides, H., & McPartland, J. (2002). Neural correlates of face recognition in young children with autism spectrum disorder, developmental delay, and typical development. *Child Development, 73,* 700–717.

Dawson, G., Jones, E. J., Merkle, K., Venema, K., Lowy, R., Faja, S., et al. (2012). Early behavioral intervention is associated with normalized brain activity in young children with autism. *Journal of the American Academy of Child and Adolescent Psychiatry, 51*(11), 1150–1159.

Dawson, G., Rogers, S., Munson, J., Smith, M., Winter, J., Greenson, J., et al. (2010). Randomized controlled trial of an intervention for toddlers with autism: The Early Start Denver Model. *Pediatrics, 123,* 1383–1391.

Dawson, G., Webb, S. J., & McPartland, J. (2005). Understanding the nature of face processing impairment in autism: Insights from behavioral and electrophysiological studies. *Developmental Neuropsychology, 27*(3), 403–424.

Diamond, A., & Lee, A. (2011). Interventions shown to aid executive function development in children 4 to 12 years old. *Science, 333,* 959–964.

DiCicco-Bloom, E., Lord, C., Zwaigenbaum, L., Courchesne, E., Dager, S. R., Schmitz, C., et al. (2006). The developmental neurobiology of autism spectrum disorder. *Journal of Neuroscience, 26*(26), 6897–6906.

Farmer, C., Thurm, A., & Grant, P. (2013). Pharmacotherapy for the core symptoms in autistic disorder: Current status of the research. *Drugs, 73,* 303–314.

Folstein, S., & Rutter, M. (1977). Infantile autism: A genetic study of 21 twin pairs. *Journal of Child Psychology and Psychiatry, 18*(4), 297–321.

Frankel, F., & Whitham, C. (2011). Parent-assisted group treatment for friendship problems of children with autism spectrum disorders. *Brain Research, 1380,* 240–245.

Frith, U. (2004). Confusions and controversies about Asperger syndrome. *Journal of Child Psychology and Psychiatry, 45,* 672–686.

Gantman, A., Kapp, S. K., Orenski, K., & Laugeson, E. A. (2012). Social skills training for young adults with high-functioning autism spectrum disorders: A randomized controlled pilot study. *Journal of Autism and Developmental Disorders, 42*(6), 1094–1103.

Gardener, H., Spiegelman, D., & Buka, S. L. (2011). Perinatal and neonatal risk factors for autism: A comprehensive meta-analysis. *Pediatrics, 128*(2), 344–355.

Grandin, T. (2009). How does visual thinking work in the mind of a person with autism?: A personal account. *Philosophical Transactions of the Royal Society B, 364*, 1437–1442.

Helt, M., Kelley, E., Kinsbourne, M., Pandey, J., Boorstein, H., Herbert, M., et al. (2008). Can children with autism recover?: If so, how? *Neuropsychology Review, 18*, 339–366.

Howlin, P., Moss, P., Savage, S., & Rutter, M. (2013). Social outcomes in mid- to later adulthood among individuals diagnosed with autism and average nonverbal IQ as children. *Journal of the American Academy of Child and Adolescent Psychiatry, 52*(6), 572–581.

Howlin, P., Savage, S., Moss, P., Tempier, A., & Rutter, M. (2014). Cognitive and language skills in adults with autism: A 40-year follow-up. *Journal of Child Psychology and Psychiatry, 55*(1), 49–58.

Kanne, S. M., Randolph, J. K., & Farmer, J. E. (2008). Diagnostic and assessment findings: A bridge to academic planning for children with autism spectrum disorders. *Neuropsychology Review, 18*, 367–384.

Kanner, L. (1943). Autistic disturbances of affective content. *Nervous Child, 2*, 217–250.

Karkhaneh, M., Clark, B., Osina, M. B., Seida, J. C., Smith, V., & Hartling, L. (2010). Social stories to improve social skills in children with autism spectrum disorder: A systematic review. *Autism, 14*, 641–662.

Kasari, C., Locke, J., Gulsrud, A., & Rotheram-Fuller, E. (2011). Social networks and friendships at school: Comparing children with and without ASD. *Journal of Autism and Developmental Disorders, 41*, 533–544.

Kenworthy, L., Anthony, L. G., Naiman, D. Q., Cannon, L., Wills, M. C., Luong-Tran, C., et al. (2014). Randomized controlled effectiveness trial of executive function intervention for children on the autism spectrum. *Journal of Child Psychology and Psychiatry, 55*(4), 374–383.

Lord, C., & Jones, R. M. (2012). Re-thinking the classification of autism spectrum disorders. *Journal of Child Psychology and Psychiatry, 53,* 490–509.

Lord, C., Petkova, E., Hus, V., Gan, W., Lu, F., Martin, D. M., et al. (2012). A multisite study of the clinical diagnosis of different autism spectrum disorders. *Archives of General Psychiatry, 69,* 306–313.

Lovaas, O. I. (1987). Behavioral treatment and normal educational and intellectual functioning in young autistic children. *Journal of Consulting and Clinical Psychology, 55,* 3–9.

Marí-Bauset, S., Zazpe, I., Mari-Sanchis, A., Llopis-González, A., & Morales-Suárez-Varela, M. (2013). Food selectivity in autism spectrum disorders: A systematic review. *Journal of Child Neurology.* Published online before print: *http://jcn.sagepub.com/content/early/2013/10/03/0883073813498821.long*

Maximo, J. O., Cadena, E. J., & Kana, R. K. (2014). The implications of brain connectivity in the neuropsychology of autism. *Neuropsychology Review, 24*(1), 1–16.

Mazefsky, C. A., McPartland, J. C., Gastgeb, H. Z., & Minshew, N. J. (2013). Comparability of DSM-IV and DSM-5 ASD research samples. *Journal of Autism and Developmental Disorders, 43,* 1236–1242.

Miller, J. N., & Ozonoff, S. (1997). Did Asperger's cases have Asperger disorder? *Journal of Child Psychology and Psychiatry, 38,* 247–251.

Narzisi, A., Muratori, F., Calderoni, S., Fabbro, F., & Urgesi, C. (2013). Neuropsychological profile in high functioning autism spectrum disorders. *Journal of Autism and Developmental Disorders, 43,* 1859–1909.

Onore, C., Careaga, M., & Ashwood, P. (2012). The role of immune dysfunction in the pathophysiology of autism. *Brain, Behavior, and Immunity, 26,* 383–392.

Ozonoff, S., Young, G. S., Carter, A., Messinger, D., Yirmiya, N., Zwaigenbaum, L., et al. (2011). Recurrence risk for autism spectrum disorders: A baby siblings research consortium study. *Pediatrics, 128*(3), e488–e495.

Politte, L. C., Henry, C. A., & McDougle, C. J. (2014). Psychopharmacological interventions in autism spectrum disorder. *Harvard Review of Psychiatry, 22*(2), 76–92.

Regier, D. A., Narrow, W. E., Clarke, D. E., Kraemer, H. C., Kuramoto,

S. J., Kuhl, E. A., et al. (2013). DSM-5 field trials in the United States and Canada: Part II. Test–retest reliability of selected categorical diagnoses. *American Journal of Psychiatry, 170,* 59–70.

Reichow, B., Steiner, A. M., & Volkmar, F. (2012). Social skills groups for people aged 6 to 21 with autism spectrum disorders. *Evidence-Based Child Health, 7,* 266–315.

Reichow, B., & Volkmar, F. R. (2010). Social skills interventions for individuals with autism: Evaluation for evidence-based practices within a best evidence synthesis framework. *Journal of Autism and Developmental Disorders, 40*(2), 149–166.

Rimland, B. (1964). *Infantile autism: The syndrome and its implications for a neural theory of behavior.* New York: Appleton-Century-Crofts.

Rogers, S. J., & Dawson, G. (2010). *The Early Start Denver Model for young children with autism: Promoting language, learning, and engagement.* New York: Guilford Press.

Rogers, S. J., Dawson G., & Vismara, L. (2012). *An early start for your child with autism.* New York: Guilford Press.

Ronemus, M., Iossifov, I., Levy, D., & Wigler, M. (2014). The role of de novo mutations in the genetics of autism spectrum disorders. *Nature Reviews Genetics, 15*(2), 133–141.

Rosti, R. O., Sadek, A. A., Vaux, K. K., & Gleeson, J. G. (2014). The genetic landscape of autism spectrum disorders. *Developmental Medicine and Child Neurology, 56*(1), 12–18.

Scahill, L., McDougle, C. J., Aman, M. G., Johnson, C., Handen, B., Bearss, K., et al. (2012). Effects of risperidone and parent training on adaptive functioning in children with pervasive developmental disorders and serious behavioral problems. *Journal of the American Academy of Child and Adolescent Psychiatry, 51*(2), 136–146.

Schipul, S. E., Keller, T. A., & Just, M. A. (2011). Inter-regional brain communication and its disturbance in autism. *Frontiers in Systems Neuroscience, 5*(10), 1–11.

Schmidt, R. J., Ozonoff, S., Hansen, R. L., Hartiala, J., Allayee, H., Schmidt, L. C., et al. (2012). Maternal periconceptional folic acid intake and risk for ASD in the CHARGE case-control study. *American Journal of Clinical Nutrition, 96,* 80–89.

Schultz, R. T., Gauthier, I., Klin, A., Fulbright, R. K., Anderson, A. W., Volkmar, F., et al. (2000). Abnormal ventral temporal cortical activity during face discrimination among individuals with autism and Asperger syndrome. *Archives of General Psychiatry, 57,* 331–340.

Shattuck, P. T., Narendorf, S. C., Cooper, B., Sterzing, P. R., Wagner, M., & Taylor, J. L. (2012). Postsecondary education and employment among youth with an autism spectrum disorder. *Pediatrics, 129,* 1042–1049.

Shelton, J. F., Tancredi, D. J., & Hertz-Picciotto, I. (2010). Independent and dependent contributions of advanced maternal and paternal ages to autism risk. *Autism Research, 3*(1), 30–39.

Siegel, M., & Beaulieu, A. A. (2012). Psychotropic medications in children with autism spectrum disorders: A systematic review and synthesis for evidence-based practice. *Journal of Autism and Developmental Disorders, 42,* 1592–1605.

Simonoff, E., Pickles, A., Charman, T., Chandler, S., Loucas, T., & Baird, G. (2008). Psychiatric disorders in children with autism spectrum disorders: Prevalence, comorbidity, and associated factors in a population-derived sample. *Journal of the American Academy of Child and Adolescent Psychiatry, 47,* 921–929.

Sparks, B. F., Friedman, S. D., Shaw, D. W., Aylward, E. H., Echelard, D., Artru, A. A., et al. (2002). Brain structural abnormalities in young children with autism spectrum disorder. *Neurology, 59*(2), 184–192.

Sterzing, P. R., Shattuck, P. T., Narendorf, S. C., Wagner, M., & Cooper, B. P. (2012). Bullying involvement and autism spectrum disorders. *Archives of Pediatric and Adolescent Medicine, 166,* 1058–1064.

Sukhodolsky, D. G., Bloch, M. H., Panza, K. E., & Reichow, B. (2013). Cognitive-behavioral therapy for anxiety in children with high-functioning autism: A meta-analysis. *Pediatrics, 132*(5), e1341–e1350.

Virues-Ortega, J., Julio, F. M., & Pastor-Barriuso, R. (2013). The TEACCH program for children and adults with autism: A meta-analysis of intervention studies. *Clinical Psychology Review, 33,* 940–953.

Volkmar, F., Reichow, B., & McPartland, J. C. (2014). *Adolescents and adults with autism spectrum disorder.* New York: Springer.

Warren, Z., McPheeters, M. L., Sathe, N., Foss-Feig, J. H., Glasser, A., et al. (2011). A systematic review of early intensive intervention for autism spectrum disorders. *Pediatrics, 127,* e1303–e1311.

Willey, L. H. (1999). *Pretending to be normal: Living with Asperger's syndrome.* London: Kingsley.

Wing, L. (1981). Asperger's syndrome: A clinical account. *Psychological Medicine, 11,* 115–129.

Wolff, J. J., Gu, H., Gerig, G., Elison, T. T., Styner, M., Gouttard, S., et al. (2012). Differences in white matter fiber tract development present from 6 to 24 months in infants with autism. *American Journal of Psychiatry, 169,* 589–600.

Index

About the Authors

Sally Ozonoff, PhD, is Endowed Professor and Vice Chair for Research in the Department of Psychiatry and the MIND Institute—a national center for the study and treatment of ASD—at the University of California, Davis. Dr. Ozonoff is widely known for her research and teaching in the areas of early diagnosis and assessment of ASD, and has an active clinical practice.

Geraldine Dawson, PhD, is Professor of Psychiatry and Director of the Duke Center for Autism and Brain Development at Duke University. She served as Founding Director of the University of Washington Autism Center. An internationally recognized autism expert with a focus on early detection, intervention, and brain plasticity in autism, Dr. Dawson is a passionate advocate for families. She is coauthor of *An Early Start for Your Child with Autism.*

James C. McPartland, PhD, is Associate Professor at the Yale Child Study Center and Director of the Yale Developmental Disabilities Clinic. He has worked with children with ASD and their families for more than 15 years. Dr. McPartland's award-winning research focuses on brain processes in ASD, with the goal of developing new approaches to diagnosis and treatment.